VISIONETICS

VISIONETICS
The Holistic Way to Better Eyesight

Lisette Scholl
with John Selby as Consultant

৯ ৶

Illustrations by Debbie Bell

A DOLPHIN BOOK
Doubleday & Company, Inc., Garden City, New York   1978

Library of Congress Cataloging in Publication Data

Scholl, Lisette.
    Visionetics.

        1. Vision disorders—Prevention.   2. Orthop-
tics.   3. Vision disorders—Psychosomatic aspects.
4. Exercise therapy.   I. Title.
RE992.07S3   617.7′5

ISBN: 0-385-13279-4
Library of Congress Catalog Card Number: 77-12882

CONTENTS

Contents

APPENDIXES

ACKNOWLEDGMENTS

I would like to extend many warm and deep thanks to:

John Selby, my soul brother and collaborator, for getting me started in the first place and for keeping me going.

Chuck Kelley and the members of the Radix staff who helped me discover and work through my fears of seeing the world around me. I also thank Chuck for broadening my knowledge on vision work and for his helpful comments on the manuscript.

Bates teacher Janet Goodrich for inspiring lessons and for convincing me that I didn't need my glasses.

Optometrist Raymond Gottlieb who spent many hours explaining the connections between brain and vision to me.

Optometrist Reg Baldwin, who may not agree with many ideas in this book, but who greatly helped me understand the physiological workings of the eyes.

My illustrator, Debbie Bell, who not only gave her all to the artwork, but also raised my spirits consistently with her infectious enthusiasm for the project and life in general.

The many friends who kept reminding me that the long hours and months of writing were worth the effort, especially Tracy and Kathy.

All of my students in vision classes and workshops. We explored unknown realms together, we peered into what seemed long, dark tunnels, and, in the end, WE SAW!

AUTHOR'S NOTE

I have used the term "holistic" frequently in this book, because it best describes my approach to vision. If you want, you can think "wholistic" when you read "holistic," and you will get a general feeling for what the word means.

The term holistic, however, from the Greek "holos," carries a very important and particular spirit, one which exemplifies the over-all mood of the holistic health movement which is growing so rapidly today. To see a human being holistically is to see that person not as an intricate neurochemical machine which can be dissected and understood because of its individual parts. Holistically, a human being is greater than the sum of its parts, being both body and spirit, mind and emotions, a unity which cannot be broken up without destroying the essence of that being.

A holistic approach to better vision, then, begins and ends with the whole being, and deals with eyesight as an integral part of that being, not as an isolated medical phenomenon. From a holistic point of view, the eyes reflect the whole being and that being's relationship with its environment. If we are to genuinely improve our eyesight, we must deal with the over-all well-being of the entire organism as well. This holistic approach is what makes this program for vision improvement work so well, allowing the personality to grow and expand as the eyesight becomes clearer.

Another preliminary note I'd like to make is that when I mention the attitudes of optometrists and ophthalmologists, I am referring to the mainstream of eye doctors. I do not include the small but growing number of professionals who are beginning to accept a holistic view of vision and to alter their practices accordingly. In this book I wish not to antagonize the established optometric community, but to encourage it to consider this alternate view of vision, and to begin to incorporate these new trends of vision retraining into their work.

If you have trouble in concentrating on the exercises without the guiding voice of a teacher, or if you would like to supplement your individual work, you may want to order some tapes of the exercises. For a brochure, contact the author at:

P.O. Box 596
Templeton, California 93465

PREFACE

In 1946 I began Bates lessons to improve my nearsighted vision. I was twenty-four years old. For the first time in fifteen years my eyes began to get better with time instead of worse. At the start I was just able to make out the largest letter on the eye chart with my better eye. This meant my acuity measured 20/200, indicating that at twenty feet I could see letters ten times normal size. My worse eye required letters twenty times normal size (20/400). After six months my eyes improved by three or four times, to 20/70. After two years the improvement was to 20/40, and I became able to pass my driver's licensing test without glasses, an achievement I have repeated eight or nine times in four different states in the intervening years. My eyes have not become 20/20 except for brief periods, but I have been able to live normally for thirty years without the eye crutches I was forced to wear throughout my childhood and youth. Nor has it been necessary for me to continue to do vision drills to keep my improvement in vision, though I have done them on occasion through the years as I felt the need.

After the great improvement in my vision, a result my ophthalmologist had assured me was impossible, I became a psychologist specializing in vision and feeling, which I found to be intimately related. With modern scientific optical equipment I demonstrated that the eyes changed optically for the better when psychologically based vision-improvement techniques were used.

But that was in the 1950s, before most people were ready for a holistic health concept of vision. In particular, people were not ready to look at the intimate association between emotion and seeing. Even Bates teachers—and my own vision improvement came from studying with fine Bates teachers—had only a limited grasp of how mental and emotional strain became translated into faulty vision.

The contribution of the present volume is that it shows this understanding. The source of the chronic tension in the eyes from which defective vision springs is blocked emotion. Knowing this provides the new key to better sight. Vision reflects our whole state of being, but particularly our emotions. Spend a relaxing day at the beach or in the mountains and chances are high that you see further, read with less strain, notice colors more vividly. Feel withdrawn or scared and note that your vision is worse. Become uptight with anger and you suffer from headache and eye strain. Refuse to cry when the painful events of life overtake you and your eyes must suffer from your locked-in tears. Let yourself feel and express openly the emotions you've been holding back, and the tensions in the eyes and body that block emotion—tensions discovered by the psychiatrist Wilhelm Reich —release and free the eyes to see.

The successful vision-improvement program frees emotions blocked in the eyes as it frees the eyes to see. The superiority of the lessons in vision improvement in this book over those written in the past comes from the author's understanding of this key point, and the incorporation of emotion-freeing exercises into her program.

So be aware as you begin your *Visionetics* program that you are working not only to improve your eyes, but at the same time (and as part of the same process) to free feelings locked in by eye tension. As you learn to see you learn to accept and express emotion that you have felt the need to block in the past. Holistic health means that no one part of the body (like the eyes) and no one function of the mind (like vision) can be treated in isolation from the rest. This book will help you deal with them as a whole.

Charles R. Kelley, Ph.D.
Director, The Radix Institute
Ojai, California

Charles R. Kelley, Ph.D., director of the Radix Institute in Southern California, is a scientist who has specialized in vision training and human factors research for twenty-five years. In 1950, he became a student of Wilhelm Reich, contributing to Reich's journals during his life and to the development of his theories since his death. He is a qualified masseur, Bates instructor, and a writer, and has served on the faculties of several universities, most recently as the George A. Miller Visiting Professor at the University of Illinois. He is a Fellow of the American Psychological Association and the Human Factors Society, and his memberships in other organizations include the International Transactional Analysis Association and the Association for Humanistic Psychology. Dr. Kelley has given Radix workshops throughout the country and abroad. Presently, his training of teachers in Radix education extends across the country, and includes both professionals and nonprofessionals.

VISIONETICS

PART ONE

CHAPTER 1

REVISIONING VISION

How to Reverse the Visual Epidemic

We are in the midst of a visual epidemic of giant proportions. Over 50 per cent of our nation's population is currently suffering from some form of vision failure which directly hinders performance and enjoyment of life. It has actually become statistically "normal" to have failing vision, and the rate of vision failure is increasing so rapidly that optometrists predict that less than 10 per cent of the population in the United States will be free of vision problems by the year 2000.

The cause of this vision failure, and the holistic approach to reversing it, is the subject of this book. Whether you are near- or farsighted, or suffer from astigmatism or poor fusion, this approach seeks to uncover the root cause of that problem and to guide you step by step to clearer vision. For those of you who have 20/20 vision, this can be a simple preventive program that will help to keep your eyesight clear throughout your life.

I personally suffered from nearsightedness, so there is naturally a slight emphasis in this book toward myopia as I discuss the causes and present exercises to alleviate poor vision. But those of you who are farsighted (hyperopic and/or presbyopic) will find almost all of the exercises as helpful to you as they are to nearsighted people. Where there is a difference in how to do an exercise depending on whether you're near- or farsighted, I will always make clear how to do the exercise to best benefit each visual problem.

The main reason for farsightedness (hyperopia) seems to be chronic muscular tension, a condition most common in many middle-aged and older people. Myopia, or nearsightedness, is the most common vision problem for young people (along with the related astigmatic and fusion problems). In middle age, a farsighted condition known as presbyopia develops, and clear sight at close range is lost.

My premise is that these different vision problems are related; that they are different manifestations of the same basic cause, chronic muscular tension. In this program I have developed exercises which deal with this general cause; the exercises specifically aim at one vision problem only in a few cases. This is why even people with "normal" vision will enjoy and benefit from the exercises as they experience the roots of their visual being.

This holistic guide to vision improvement blends several self-help techniques which I have found to have a positive effect on sight; but the foundation of the exercises is drawn from a technique known as the Bates method. Dr. William Bates, an ophthalmologist who practiced in New York around the turn of this century, postulated that the key to clear vision was a relaxed, coordinated effort of mind and body. He challenged the orthodox view that vision is a mechanical process controlled primarily by the random forces of heredity. Bates also found that vision fluctuated according to mood and circumstance, sometimes radically. This finding also countered orthodox opinion, which saw vision as unaffected by either an individual's health, mood, or his environment. Bates believed that as a result of mental tension, the muscles surrounding the eyes contracted so much that they forced the eyeball out of its proper shape or alignment. When the tension was relieved, he said, the eyes returned to their natural shape, coordination between mind and eye was regained, and sight became clear. Bates devised a series of mental and physical exercises that proved astoundingly successful in reducing and even "curing" the problems of nearsightedness, farsightedness, and astigmatism.

However, the Bates method used alone has had as many failures as successes, primarily because Bates did not see more fully into the role of emotions on vision. Certain discoveries in the field of psychiatry were necessary to understand the specific relationship between kinds of tension and their visual manifestations. The pioneering work was done by Dr. Wilhelm Reich, a colleague of Freud's. Like Bates, Reich's work was too controversial to be accepted during his lifetime, but it is now accepted as the foundation for all the modern mind/body approaches to physical and mental health. Reich found that specific emotional reactions resulted in specific bodily contractions. Bands of chronic muscular tension are created, which remain locked in the body even after the real cause for the reaction is long gone. These bands of tension block the free and natural flow of energy through the body, and the individual is left with impaired physical and emotional capabilities. What began as the body protecting itself by contracting against emotional pain ends up as a condition in which the body lessens its ability to feel good, or to feel much at all.

Visually, this means that the muscles in and around the eyes are related to emotional states in the body. When the visual system is confronted by realities an individual would emotionally prefer not to see, the brain can send a message to the eyes to do just that, not see. We all do this every day to some extent—there are days we see and feel well, and days we see and feel poorly. However, if the source of the stress is not alleviated for a long period, the eyes may lose their flexibility, and vision becomes impaired. Still, regarding our eyes as highly sensitive parts of the whole being, we can do specific exercises which bring about relaxation of the eye muscles, integrate the visual organs with the visual areas of the brain, and allow for the recovery of spontaneous visual health, while also encouraging over-all personal growth and emotional well-being.

When I began retraining my eyes, I felt threatened by the thought that responses to experiences in my past could have caused my loss of clear vision. I felt that I was being asked to take the blame for my poor vision. The optometrist I went to had never even hinted that I had anything to do with my vision failure. How could anyone suggest that how my eyes functioned was related to how I felt emotionally, or to how I had reacted to my environment in the past?

However, I began to realize that there certainly was much in my past that I literally did not want to see, that I chose not to see. And once I made this realization, a whole new world of hope and growth opened up to me. Just as I had once chosen not to see, I could now choose again to see. My eyes, after all, were an outgrowth of my brain itself, with brain cells making up the sense organs in the retina. I realized that in desiring to improve my vision, I was really desiring to grow as a person, to overcome basic reactions which had resulted in my closing down one of my sense organs, and to again see the world clearly, openly, holistically.

From a historical or evolutionary point of view, it is obvious why so many of us are victims of the visual epidemic. Our culture is suffering from a general level of tension and stress unheard of fifty years ago. Future shock is virtually universal as an emotional condition in the civilized world. The pace of life has speeded up to the point where few of us can keep pace with the advancing technology which more and more seems to determine our fate. As we have lost our sense of self-sufficiency, we have naturally grown more apprehensive and anxious about our well-being and our future. And having the threat of nuclear holocaust hanging over our heads every second of our lives can only generate anxiety.

In addition, all of us inevitably encounter emotional situations which can result in the body's reacting with a physical illness or weakness. Ulcers, heart attacks, high blood pressure, and perhaps even cancer are often associated with chronic blocking of emotions which, when not allowed expression, generate a physical symptom to express the inner trauma. And it is a growing opinion of many experts in the vision field that such emotional traumas, usually in childhood, can bring about loss of clear vision.

Unfortunately, glasses do not "cure" the problem at all. In fact, they distort vision: Seeing through glass is just not the same as seeing without glasses. However, this problem is minor when compared to the long-term effects of wearing glasses. If you break your leg and have it in a cast, the leg muscles atrophy so that it is difficult to walk normally again when the cast is removed. This is exactly what corrective lenses do: They inhibit the free-flowing muscular work of the eye muscles, and do the work for them, so that when you take your glasses off, your vision is even worse than before you got the glasses.

Dependence on and need for corrective lenses afflict over 50 per cent of us in this country. If 50 per cent were suffering from a strange disease which forced us to depend on crutches all the time, we would have solved the problem long before now. But eyeglasses have been tolerated and often even praised, although they are, in reality, prescription drugs which relieve the symptom just as a painkiller would relieve the pain of an ulcer. They do nothing to cure the problem underlying the symptom; in fact, they almost always make the problem worse. This is obviously not a sane way to deal with an epidemic.

The program in this book does not offer an instant "cure," nor is it an effortless one. But it will take you step by step toward better and better vision, to the point where you can probably throw away your glasses as you return to a more natural visual state. If you will just spend as much time helping your eyes as you do brushing your teeth and cleaning your house, changing your car's oil or jogging to keep fit, there is no reason why your vision can't become independent of glasses and remain that way for the rest of your life.

And not only will your vision improve, your whole world view will improve along with it—they are integrally woven, and improving one cannot help but improve the other. As you come to understand your sense of vision, you will gain deep insights into your personality and into how you perceive the world. And as your visual perception expands, so will your appreciation of the world around you.

As you will notice, many of the exercises are not even directly focused on the eyes as such, but deal with the whole body. These exercises are designed to aid circulation and to increase the general energy level of the body as they help reduce anxiety and chronic muscular tension. Much emphasis is placed on relaxation, both physically and mentally, for if the body is constricted, the muscles around your eyes are most likely in chronic tension. Coordination is also a vital factor in vision retraining, and this coordination will be augmented by general body awareness. I have also drawn from such diverse traditions as Hathayoga, Tantric Buddhist meditations, hypnotic suggestion, and the emotional-release exercises of Wilhelm Reich and his followers, in addition to some standard optometric exercises, and

7

many of Bates's techniques. Whenever I found insight and concrete suggestions which worked, I have incorporated them into the program I used to bring my vision back to an independent, comfortable state, and which I later taught to my students, with similar success.

Before presenting the program itself, I will briefly discuss how the eyes work, how the brain integrates the inputs from the eyes to give us our perception of sight, and how different emotional and environmental factors can alter our perception and create poor vision. Some technical understanding of how your eyes work will give you a sound foundation upon which to build your visual rehabilitation program.

Also included is my own Eyelogue, a journal of my day-by-day experiences as I went through this program. I encourage you to also keep such a journal, and offer you mine, to give you an idea of what to expect and as a framework which you may want to use in your own journal.

There are twenty sessions in the program, and I recommend that you read the whole book through once before you start the program itself. This is not a vital step in the process, but it will afford you a good overview. Then, as you go through the program step by step from start to finish, I recommend that you spend two days on each session. This doubles the program length, but insures that you have integrated the exercises fully; and, more importantly, this approach makes the program more comfortable and easy for your eyes and body so that there is no pressure or strain. If you would like to spend even more time with each individual session before moving on to the next, so much the better. Once you have completed the program you will understand your individual visual needs and problems, and can design your own program. In the back of this book are some sample exercise schedules to adapt and use accordingly.

How much you can expect your vision to improve and how long it will take depends on how long you have worn glasses, how poor your sight is at present, and on your own attitude. If you are committed to change and are able to give approximately forty-five minutes to an hour per day to the exercises, your vision will improve in about two months' time. This is an "average" improvement which tends to hold, for example, with myopes no worse than 20/200 at the start; 20/200 means that a letter must be ten times the normal size to be seen clearly.

Vision usually improves quickly in the first two months and then reaches a temporary plateau. The farther you have to go to bring your sight to an acceptable, independent level, the longer your vision may hold at each plateau. If your sight improves, for example, from 20/200 to 20/100 in a two-month period, you may then find that even if you continue to exercise with the same intensity you still may not see much more improvement for the following two months. Then, usually, another spurt of growth and change will occur. So that you won't get discouraged by the plateau, I suggest that when you reach it you decrease your concentrated efforts down to a minimal schedule (say, from a one-hour plan to a twenty-minute plan) and just enjoy the amount of success you have achieved thus far.

If your vision problems are moderate, you will probably join the minority of those able to return to actual 20/20 acuity. However, even a 50 per cent improvement in your eyesight, together with new visual habits and different attitudes, should make most of you largely independent from a need for corrective lenses. Personally, I have thus far changed the way I see to the point where I am comfortable and functional without glasses about 80 per cent of the time. During the remaining 20 per cent I am realistic about my situation, as I hope you will be, and wear glasses.

This whole program is really about change. Much of it will be a matter of gently easing your muscles and habits out of their old tense ways. If you feel your physical and environmental living conditions still contribute to your poor sight, you may have to make a considerable change in life-style to effect the change in your sight. If you discover that you had emotional reasons for not wanting to see, you have to be willing to confront and deal with those feelings. Any or all of these changes may be in store for you. Let them evolve naturally, in their own good time, rather than pushing for them. Trying to force change you are not ready for at the moment will only create tension, which, of course, will in turn create poor vision.

The Zen masters call the attempt to force change "pushing the river." Don't push your river, but help it flow as it needs to. I wish your sight a speedy recovery, but I have seen too many people set back their progress by trying too hard. Let the world out there gradually come back into your scope of vision—don't attempt to grab for it. It comes like sleep, when you are relaxed and no longer looking for it. Allow yourself and your eyes the time and space they need in which to grow, and enjoy yourself during every step of your journey.

CHAPTER 2

MOVING BEYOND THE OLD WAYS

The Six Myths of Optometry

To approach the nature of sight from a holistic point of view, we must overcome certain traditional beliefs which stand in the way of vision recovery. The field of optometry has provided us with a considerable amount of invaluable research, and it has been helpful in establishing the use of corrective lenses for certain visual problems. However, corrective lenses are not the answer for everyone—visual retraining can help many people to do without glasses for much of the time, and a few people will be able to throw away their glasses altogether. The first step in acquiring a new way of seeing is to take a close look at the practices and goals of optometry. There are six myths perpetrated by this profession, of which we should all be aware.

The first myth insists that it is impossible for the eyes to recover their natural sight. Almost every optometrist in the country imbues his patients with this sense of hopelessness, so that many people actually expect their vision to deteriorate, as if that were its natural tendency. The truth of the matter is that your eyes will indeed grow worse if you believe they are supposed to, but you can reverse the trend. If people can recover from heart attacks by exercising, why not expect a similar response from eye exercise? The trouble is that eye doctors still cling to the myth of inevitable vision failure, and therefore cannot or do not prescribe remedies for vision recovery.

A second myth propagated by the optometric profession is that of

20/20 vision. This myth was created arbitrarily so as to give some statistical "norm" to vision, although 20/20 vision makes sense only in relation to corrective lenses. When this figure is said to represent "normal" vision, it implies that our vision is a static constant which maintains a particular sharpness at all times. It implies that we all see the same way, that we all conform to the norm established by the optometric profession, whose business it is to find fault with our vision. This 20/20 myth is perhaps the most insidious one when it comes to revisioning vision, because it has conditioned us to believe there is a "right" way to see.

In actuality, nothing could be further from the truth. We are all unique individuals. We have unique voices, unique bodies, unique minds. So why shouldn't we have a unique way of seeing the world? And why should we alter our unique vision for a norm imposed on us from the outside? This is particularly important when we consider children's vision. To take a child whose vision is not normal and to slap glasses on the child whether or not he or she wants glasses is to violate that child's integrity at a deep level. It is saying to the child that the child's perception of the world is not right. Imagine how this affects the child's personality at that time?

There is an antiquated doctrine behind the 20/20 myth, which states that the shape of the eyeball does not change in response to environmental and emotional inputs; that the eyeball is an isolated organ which does not respond to other changes in the body. And it concludes that one's vision does not change regularly as one's emotions change, that one's vision is a constant rather than a variable.

It is easy to understand why the optometric profession is still caught up in this antiquated version of how the eyes work. Optometrics evolved out of a purely mechanical science, optics. Optics does not deal with the human body at all; its concern is with the refraction of light. As such, optics as a science is not adequate for dealing with the health of the visual sense organs. There is now ample scientific evidence to support a new theory, that the eyes are extremely sensitive emotional organs. It has been proven that when threatened with an electric shock, one's eyes go temporarily nearsighted. And when one is confronted with a new visual scene, eyesight temporarily goes blurry until the brain relays the message to the eyes.

Another optometric myth is that you will ruin your eyes if you don't wear your glasses. This idea has disastrous effects on children, because it forces them to develop a dependency on that which will cause more harm to their eyes. The truth is, the more you wear your glasses, the less chance you have of spontaneously recovering your natural vision. In this program I will be encouraging you to go without your glasses as much as you can.

Yet another optometric myth is that you will ruin your eyes through too much close-up work. However, the problem with close work is actually the stress which in most cases accompanies that work. When we force ourselves to read for hours a laboriously detailed text, we often develop tension in the eyes and head. If we are reading an exciting novel for the same length of time, we almost never develop any tension in the eyes. The reason is that vision is designed to work freely, to be an effortless experiencing of our environment. Chronic anxiety and overwork force the eyes beyond a comfortable point, when the body is actually tensing in response—and this in turn affects the way we see.

A myth which I have discussed earlier should be mentioned again. In optometrics there is no accepted relationship between vision and personality. But psychological studies have found, as we shall see later, that there are very definite personality and body types associated with particular vision problems, and growth in personality very often causes growth in vision.

The sixth and final myth that optometrists would have us believe is that vision fails as we grow older, due to a gradual hardening of the lens of the eye. This is presently true; most older people do have to wear glasses to see clearly. But why does this happen? Is it simply a matter of the body giving up? Once we look at aging from a holistic point of view, we can see causes for vision failure which are not purely physiological, and we can see ways of avoiding such vision failure as we grow older. Being "old" is often a state of mind. The key to maintaining clear eyesight into old age is to remain flexible, open to your environment, and expressive of your emotions. And it is never too late to begin improving your health and your vision.

So we have the old myths which lead to hopelessness and a continuation of the vision epidemic, and we have the new truths which offer hope. The eyes are not static organs, and the possibility of correcting your poor vision is not hopeless. With new ways of thinking, which more adequately reflect the potential as well as the realities of vision, we can achieve success where optometrists would predict failure.

Because we must come to a new understanding of the eye and its relationship to the rest of the body, we need to take a fresh look at the physical aspects of visual perception. In the next chapter I will discuss how the eyes function, and how tension and poor seeing habits influence eyesight.

CHAPTER 3

A LOOK INSIDE YOUR EYES

You See With Your Brain

Vision is a team sport; it takes two to play. It takes light from the sun or an artificial source, and it takes a receptive nervous system stimulated by that light energy. Together, light and life create vision.

Vision seems quite miraculous when we consider the fact that we don't really see the object, but rather the light reflecting off the object's surface. Most objects absorb only certain wave lengths of light and reject others; for instance, if an object absorbs red, it reflects blue, and we see that object as blue. If an object is totally black, it absorbs all the light striking it, and we experience only the absence of light. In a very real sense, we see the opposite quality of that object, not the quality it contains.

Let's follow the light reflected off an object as it enters the eye. Light first penetrates the clear, curved surface of the eye called the cornea. The curvature of the cornea—together with that of the lens—bends the incoming light so that the rays converge on the retina, the rear surface of the eye, where the image is recorded and sent to the brain. The shape of the cornea is critical; if it is misshapen, the light will be scattered instead of striking the retina on the precise spot where clear, detailed vision takes place. The image will be distorted rather than clean and clear. The condition in which the cornea is curved elliptically like a football rather than round like a basketball (the normal cornea shape) is called astigmatism.

Visionetics

We all have a certain degree of astigmatism. This is why we see stars in the sky and automobile headlights in the distance as radiating rather than as perfectly uniform light sources. The amount of astigmatism can change from moment to moment, from day to day, depending on environment and circumstances. The following quick exercise will give you an idea of how much astigmatism is affecting your eyes at this moment.

All of the lines and circles in the first illustration below are of equal blackness. However, if your cornea is not optimally shaped, you'll see one or more of the circles darker than the others (the horizontal lines will be in focus, but the vertical lines will be blurred, or vice versa). In the second illustration, astigmatism is present if you see any pie-shaped areas as lighter than the rest of the form. Take note of how you saw each illustration, and go back to this page later: You will probably notice that your astigmatism will increase or decrease.

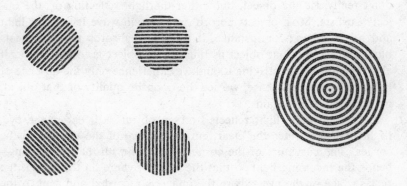

The cornea is made up of living cells, but there are no blood vessels running through the cornea to nourish these cells; the same is true of the lens. Instead, the cornea and the lens are fed by the liquid which adjoins them: the aqueous humor. This liquid is secreted and absorbed by the body every four hours, feeding the cornea while maintaining the pressure necessary to sustain its proper curvature.

Light intensity is controlled at this point by the iris and the pupil. The iris muscles both contract and expand in a circular direction and open or close the pupil to adjust to the intensity of the light source. Pupils react in this manner not only to light, but also to emotion. When a person is suddenly frightened, his irises open wide; when he or she is angry, the iris will narrow somewhat. In the fear response of the wide-open pupil, distance vision is reduced, and with the pupil narrower, distance vision is increased. These responses parallel the general body responses to such emotions as fear when the body is paralyzed and freezes. Anger, on the other hand, is a reaction which prepares most people for action, including good eyesight for that action. Myopic, or nearsighted, people react to anger with wide-open pupils, and farsighted people tend to narrow their pupils in anger.

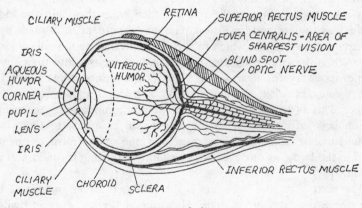

(a) Parts of the eye

Light passes through the hole of the pupil and encounters the lens, which has the primary function of adjusting the focus of the light for near- or far-distance viewing. The lens increases its curvature for viewing near objects, a function known as accommodation. As I mentioned earlier, the lens receives its nourishment for growth from the aqueous humor separating it from the cornea. Because the lens grows from the inside out, like an onion, building up cells on the outside, the inner cells can die due to lack of nutrients. This often causes the lens to harden, and presbyopia often develops, a condition optometrists claim is inevitable to middle-aged and/or older people.

After passing through the lens, the light continues through another jellylike substance which fills the eye behind the lens. It is called the vitreous humor, a liquid which maintains the shape of the eyeball against the eye muscles. This liquid is not replaced by the body, so that if it is lost, the eye collapses. If there is debris in the vitreous humor, the individual will be bothered by harmless but annoying "floaters," or "spots before the eyes." This can sometimes be remedied by relaxation and proper nutrition.

Sight is an active process, requiring effort of the eye muscles which control the shape of the lens. These muscles, called ciliary muscles, play a key part in how well our eyes function, as they shift the focus of the lens to near and far vision. The lens is suspended in place by a transparent membrane, which in turn is controlled by the ciliary muscles. When the ciliary muscles tense, the lens springs into the convex shape necessary for near vision. This is accommodation. When the ciliary muscles relax, the lens flattens, allowing for distance, or far, vision. This is called the relaxation of accommodation. Accommodation is a critical factor in the way our eyes adjust to the world around us. In fact, the ciliary muscle is one of the most frequently used in the body, as our eyes are constantly adjusting for near and far vision.

The next place the light hits is the retina, the rear surface of the eye where the "seeing" is done. However, if there is a great deal of tension in the muscles surrounding the eyes, the extraocular muscles surrounding the retina actually squeeze the eyeball out of its proper shape, making it too long or too short. When this happens the refracted image is focused in front of or behind the retina instead of directly on it, and the image is blurry.

There are two sets of muscles controlling the shape and movement of the eyes. The recti muscles stretch from front to back, and the ob-

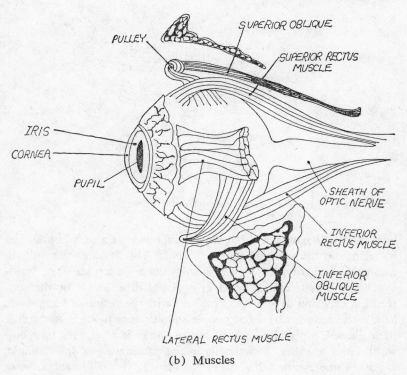

(b) Muscles

lique muscles belt the eyeball in a circular manner. If the recti are pulled up tight in a state of chronic tension, the eyeball will become shortened, the image will land behind the retina, and the resulting vision is called hyperopic, or farsighted. If the obliques are tightly squeezing the eye, the eyeball becomes elongated, the image falls in front of the retina, and the individual is myopic, or nearsighted.

Malfunctioning of the extraocular muscles can also result in problems with image fusion. This is caused when the muscles in each eye do not pull together with equal force, and a slightly different image is recorded in each eye. Normally, the brain can fuse the two images

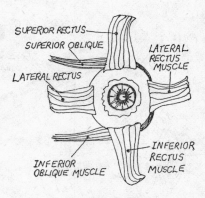

(c) Muscles, frontal view

into one single image, without any strain, but after a certain point, an imbalance in the working muscles occurs. This imbalance results in headaches and gritty, achy eyes, or even worse, in crossed eyes, "wall-eyes" (eyes that turn outward in opposite directions), or the suppression of vision in one eye. Problems with the fusion of images can be the one reason why a few people should be cautious in discarding their glasses, especially early in vision work. If your eyes turn outward, cross or differ dramatically in their strength (as, for example, 20/50 in one eye and 20/200 in the other), you will want to work often with each eye individually to insure the health of both.

Meanwhile, if the cornea, lens, and extraocular muscles have been working correctly, the image will finally land on the retina. This back layer of the eye is made up of photosensitive brain cells known as rods and cones. When the image hits the retina it is actually recorded upside down, but the brain interprets it right side up. The rods are the recorders of black and white colors and gross shapes; they also account for peripheral vision. The cones see colors and enable us to detect small objects and details.

Most of the cones are located in a tiny spot near the center of the retina, called the fovea. The fovea is the place where the light and the images it carries must converge if sight is to have the sharp clarity of

20/20 vision. The fovea operates effectively only when the visual image is continuously and rapidly shifted—normally, this movement is natural and unconscious.

So far I have concentrated on the purely physical aspects of how our eyes work, although there is much more to sight than the physical structure and functioning of the eyes. There are also natural, unconscious habits of seeing which in the presence of tension cease to work properly, with visual acuity suffering as a result. These habits are scanning, breathing, and blinking.

Scanning is a function of the eye that occurs without any conscious awareness when there is no tension, and, therefore, no effort in our seeing. We do not see entire scenes or even objects in one all-encompassing look. We see, as Aldous Huxley described in *The Art of Seeing,* in analytical, piecemeal form. The normally functioning eye scans a scene with a constant rapid, jerky motion. All the bits of information picked up during the scanning are sent to the brain, and is then "seen" as a whole.

When emotional tension enters the scene, the scanning response freezes up. The individual strains his eyes to compensate, and vision becomes even worse. Making a conscious effort to see is an unnatural act and results in trying to "take in" the whole scene at once. Fortunately, through the use of exercises and relaxation techniques, the scanning mechanism can be reactivated. Even without practicing any other exercises, many people have found great improvement in the visual abilities simply through learning to keep their eyes constantly moving in a subtle, relaxed manner.

The way we breathe and blink also has enormous impact on our sight. The moment we freeze and tense against an experience, our breathing and blinking become inhibited, and so does our ability to see clearly. Since there is so little actual blood supply to our eyes, most nourishment must be gained through oxygen, and vision can suffer when normal breathing becomes jagged or inhibited.

When we don't blink we don't supply the corneal surface with moisture. The normal blinking rate of about three times every ten seconds keeps the eyes wet, smoothed, and soothed with momentary periods of darkness. Unblinking eyes quickly become dry, tired, and strained, and sight is affected. Like scanning and normal breathing, natural blinking can be relearned so that the eye's potential is greatly enhanced.

For a long time it was thought that vision failure was simply bad luck due to an inherent weakness in the organ itself. This thinking is changing, just as we have had to change our thinking about the causes of such illnesses as heart disease, cancer, high blood pressure, asthma, and pneumonia, to name a few. Our attitudes and emotions seem to be what govern our response to stress factors, along with certain environmental or hereditary tendencies.

Visual problems, just like most other major diseases, can be correlated to certain emotions, as well as to certain personality types. William Bates used the term "mental tension" to describe the most common reason for many types of refractive error. More recently, the work of psychologists and researchers such as Young, Rosanes, and Kelley has resulted in a clearer portrait of what kind of person suffers what kind of visual problem.

There is a tendency, for example, for nearsighted people to be shy, rather introspective, somewhat stubborn and inflexible, often lost in thoughts and daydreams, and sometimes uncomfortable with others. They tend to try to avoid confrontations with others and to have a high stress tolerance. Physically, myopes are prone to being underactive, having soft bodies, weak legs, a tense depressed chest, and a husky, breathy voice. They carry a great deal of tension in the throat, chest, back of head, jaws, and scalp. In terms of past or present emotional reactions to situations, nearsighted people are either fearful, or they make a great effort not to admit to fears. This in turn makes it difficult for them to express or feel anger as well.

Hyperopes, on the other hand, have been found to be extroverted and rather aggressive; they sometimes exhibit behavior problems at home and at school, are aware of their environment rather than off in daydreams, and are more easily influenced by others. Physically, they are often active, sometimes to the point of hyperactivity, have hard stiff bodies with chests overexpanded rather than underexpanded, and they carry much chronic tension around the eyes, the sides of the neck, and the back. Emotionally, anger and rage, especially from past experiences, are suppressed.

Severe astigmatism problems have not been as thoroughly researched, but I have found with my students, as have many optometrists with their patients, that a high proportion of people with a great deal of astigmatism were often children who changed schools often or who experienced many family upheavals. Also, newly arrived immigrants from vastly different cultures often suffer from astigmatism. The distortion of astigmatism seems to imply that the individuals at some point in their lives suffered a sense of confusion and disorientation, rather than a more directed response of fear or anger.

Even presbyopia, the loss of accommodation associated with middle and old age, which usually requires reading glasses, seems to have certain psychological implications. The more active the individuals, the more zest they have for life and the better physical care they take of themselves, hardening of the lens may occur much later. If growing old is not accepted, and the individual inhibits the characteristic hyperopic feelings of anger, it may well be that the visual system responds to help blur out this undesirable view of the self.

At the psychological core of each of these visual types is a desire, at some level, not to see. Basically, this is just our organism's way of protecting itself from emotional trauma. The stress or trauma can be anything from intense family problems to a feeling of being overwhelmed by our modern-day living environment.

The body's natural, protective response to threat has, unfortunately, been "helped" by the miracles of modern science. Corrective lenses create a situation where the eyes cannot see clearly unless they remain adjusted to the glasses. If you've ever tried on a pair much too strong for you, you know the eyes are greatly strained in that situation; and, of course, the more the function of seeing is done by glasses instead of by our eyes themselves, the more they simply weaken from disuse. Additionally, from my own experience and that of many others, it appears that when the emotional desire not to see a threatening environment is still present, while glasses provide a clarity in spite of that desire, our eyes may continue to try to protect us from the view by tensing up in an attempt to shut out the sight of the threat.

In my work I have been constantly encouraged by the vast numbers of people also searching for a way out of this growing dilemma. I believe we are going to do it. The eyes and their workings are still mysterious; there is still no guaranteed method for quickly or easily bringing our sight back, but the program outlined in this book includes most of the successful methods being used today. Why some of them work as well as they do may seem technologically impossible, but the fact is that they do work. How well they work is up to you as an individual. The key lies in having a positive belief that you can change, and in wanting that change intensely.

Perhaps the most important advice I can offer you, however, is not to worry about 20/20 vision. If you push for it, it will always allude you. Concentrate, instead, on what you do see. Astoundingly, so many of us with poor sight are so upset at not seeing clearly that we don't even appreciate or use what we do see. If you start with the goal of making the most of what you already perceive, you'll find rapid and fulfilling progress in store for you. This will come from relearning what I've referred to as "habits of seeing." With these natural and proper habits you'll greatly increase your visual strength and independence, even if you don't complete the program of exercises. Once you become aware of what Huxley so aptly called the "art" of seeing, you'll begin to see much better than you do presently.

Give yourself time. Patience, love, and a positive attitude toward your whole self and the whole world you want to see are all important. That's why this is the "holistic" guide.

PART TWO

THE EXERCISES

Now you're ready to begin the exercises. There are twenty exercise sessions in this program, and each exercise consists of three parts: the Whole-body exercises, the Eye Warm-ups, and the Main Event. I recommend that you begin with a brief reading of the program before actually following it through in the sequence presented. You should spend two days on each session, so that your first time through the program should take about four to six weeks. Then you may turn to the sample exercise schedules at the back of this book, and design your own schedule according to your individual needs. You can choose one of these sample schedules or structure one of your own, but keep in mind that you'll need at least an hour a day, broken up into two or three periods, to see a 50 per cent or more improvement in your eyesight. Whenever you do the exercises is up to you. Some people find that what works best for them is ten minutes in the morning, ten minutes in the afternoon, and thirty to forty minutes later in the day, after work or before bedtime.

Generally, there's no way to overdo. You can indulge in most of these exercises for as long as you like; the only ones to do in moderation are the whole-body exercises—if they tire you—and some variations of the vision exercises known as Accommodation and Fusion, which give the eyes a strenuous workout. If you become ill or excessively tired, don't do any exercises requiring effort of the eyes. When you're sick, also try to avoid reading; at these times the best thing you can do for your eyes is the relaxing exercises known as Palming.

The exercises improve your eyesight in seven different, but related, ways. Each of the seven groups of exercises has a slightly different role, which builds upon and enhances the effects of the others. The most general group of exercises draws upon the whole body for a subtle improvement in all of your body systems. Whatever it is your body needs: improved muscle tone, increased energy, improved circulation, muscular relaxation, even emotional release—you'll find an exercise for it here. The other six areas of concentration are specifically directed at the eyes.

Palming and Visualization exercises will relax the eye muscles and the mind, and will develop your ability to see clearly with your mind's eye, a crucial prerequisite to physically clear sight.

The exercises done in the sunlight will also relax the mind and the eye muscles. Additionally, the eyes will receive vital nutrition from the sun's rays, which stimulate the whole system as well as the eyes themselves. If you are overly sensitive to the sun, these exercises will gradually rid you of that problem.

The fourth basic area of work will be in the skill known as Accommodation. This is the eye's ability to shift focus from near to far. Whether you are near- or farsighted, this is crucial to sight improvement. If you are presbyopic ("old age" sight) this is probably the most important area for you, together with whole-body exercises. However, these exercises can cause strain if you overdo them, so be sure to follow the directions to rest afterward.

The Fusion exercises should also always be followed by a good rest period so that your work is not negated by strain. These exercises will retrain your eye muscles so that they align both eyes on the same spot at the same time. Even if your eye problems are slight you should make good use of these exercises, as fusion trouble tends to precede and accompany all other vision problems.

The sixth exercise group is called Centralization and Mobility. Centralization is the method we'll use to retrain the eyes to utilize the fovea, the central point of sight, with better accuracy and ease. Mobility goes hand in hand with centralization, as it is the ability to keep the eyes effortlessly moving and sending information to the brain rather than remaining locked in a frozen stare.

Last, we'll be doing a lot of Swinging. Swinging exercises relax the whole body, ease the eye muscles out of their tension, and loosen the visual system so that it can again work with agility and freedom.

I'll gradually introduce all seven groups of exercises in the twenty sessions. If lack of time or any personal factors prevent you from doing them in the order given, you won't be negating your over-all efforts. However, the sequence of the exercises enables each one to build upon the last, thus giving you maximum return on your work. At the back of the book you'll find a handy listing of all the exercises, broken down into these seven groups.

The first part of each exercise session is called "Whole-body Exercises." Sight is such an integral part of our whole physical make-up that many people, especially myopes, have found that undergoing an intense postural retraining program, such as the Alexander method, has had a profound impact on their visual capabilities. The body exercises will not only improve your posture but also increase circulation, enliven the heart, tone and strengthen the whole body, and promote the integration of the mind, body, and emotions. Your vision is greatly affected by your bodily fitness, and each physical exercise presented here has been chosen for its relationship to sight. Do the whole-body exercises—as well as *all* of the exercises—without your glasses.

The second part of each session is called "Eye Warm-ups." Don't let the term "warm-up" let you slip into skipping this section. These are vital exercises, not supplementary fillers. Even if they are short, simple, or have been presented before, it's crucial to include them in your schedule.

The third part of your workout is "The Main Event." This is the meatiest section of the session, the one which should occupy most of your time and concentration. Later on in the program many of these main events will become warm-ups, but they are introduced with so much emphasis because it is so important to learn them thoroughly.

Following each exercise session you'll find a page or two of tips and reminders about how to use the exercises throughout the day. I'll also be giving you information about how various factors in our everyday surroundings affect eyesight, and how you can counteract (or take advantage of) some of these. This section is called "In Between," because it deals with things you can do for your eyesight throughout the day, not just at exercise times. In many ways, the information you'll find in this In Between section is at least as important as the exercises, because it will help you to develop new visual habits which you can carry throughout the rest of your life.

The final and crucial part of the program is "Your Eyelogue," which is a personal journal of your successes, failures, insights, and fears as you progress through the exercises. I think you'll discover that the Eyelogue is an invaluable source of feedback, and you may find that keeping a journal can be the best means, short of "professional" help, of exploring how emotional and environmental factors have contributed to the way you now see. This written record can also function as an exercise of sorts, as you flip back through the pages occasionally, to review your progress or gain a different perspective on a particular exercise. I've included, at the back of this book, several selections from my own Eyelogue, to share my experiences with you.

So off you go, on a journey of visual change and growth. Stick to the program, but don't push it. You are going to learn a great deal about the way you now see, and how you came to see this way. Then, little by little, you—and your eyesight—are going to change, for the better. Indulge in the exercises; get to know and enjoy your entire being. As all the sensations of joy, exploration, curiosity, and relaxation come to you, you'll know you're making progress.

SESSION ONE

a. Whole-body Exercises

Let's begin with a general exercise to wake up the whole being and release tension from the body. One of the finest, and also the most instinctual, exercises for increased circulation and muscular relaxation is simple stretching. No self-respecting animal would ever begin its day without indulging in a whole-body stretch, but we often never

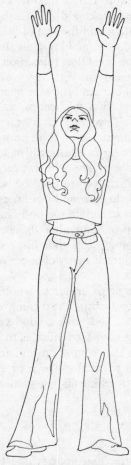

Whole-body Stretch

break out of our morning stiffness and sluggishness, and our eyes reflect this.

Yawning is a small quick stretch, so let's do it first. Just drop your jaw, close your eyes, and take a deep breath. Feel your tongue tense, your face muscles tighten, and the rest of your body become taut with energy. Then exhale slowly, making a sighing sound with your voice as you discharge tension and allow relaxation to fill your body.

Notice what happened to your eyes after a few yawns. They stretched, too, didn't they? And the tear ducts were stimulated so that your eyes received that vital lubrication they need regularly to stay healthy. If you blink a few times after yawning you may notice that your vision improves temporarily. Every time you yawn, look for this improvement. The more you are sensitive to such improvement and encourage it, the faster your eyes will recover.

We tend to yawn when we are tired or bored. This is because our breathing has become sluggish and our energy level low, and a yawn is an automatic way to stimulate the body back to a relaxed but alert state. I encourage you to remember to yawn many times each day. Just think about yawning, drop your jaw and inhale; usually a yawn will come out. Give yourself many chances during the day to perform this basic quick stretch.

To take the yawn a step further to whole-body exercise, stand up and leisurely reach up toward the ceiling or sky with both hands. Close your eyes, inhale, and have a good yawn, sighing as loudly as you want and allowing your face muscles to make a squinting expression. Then relax with the exhalation and feel the energy starting to flow in your body, and particularly in your eyes. Go ahead and spend the next few minutes stretching all you want!

b. Eye Warm-ups

Now that you've stretched your whole body, how do your eyes feel? How is your vision today? Did you do the stretching with your glasses on or off? In general, how much of the day do you wear corrective lenses? Some of you will be going through these sessions even if you don't wear glasses, but most of you do, so begin to be aware of your glasses in front of your eyes when you're wearing them. Experiment by taking them off in different situations to see how you feel without them. The more you face your blur and begin to relate to it, the quicker you will be able to clear up that blur.

Right now, take off your glasses and look off into the distance if you're nearsighted, or close up if you're farsighted. Examine your blur. What does it look like out there? How do you feel inside when looking into your blur? Do you feel comfortable not having to see what's out there, or does it make you feel anxious?

While you're still looking at your blur, focus your attention to your breathing. Is it shallow or deep? Is it regular or does it catch somewhere as you hold your breath? Don't do anything to alter your breathing, just be aware of how you breathe when confronting your blur. Later we will help you correct any bad habits which shut down your breathing and thus rob your entire system of oxygen and energy. For now, just begin to observe your normal breathing habits. Our breathing is one of our most sensitive parts when considering how emotions affect the body. People with poor vision almost always have poor breathing habits, and we will explore why this is so and what to do to correct it.

Now focus on whether or not you are blinking regularly as you look off into your blur. Not blinking is another bad habit common to those with poor vision. The normal eye blinks an average of three times every ten seconds. The blinks are light, quick, effortless, which lubricate the eyeball. Be aware of how often you normally blink, and if your blinks are tense or relaxed.

While still looking at your blur, try to determine if your body is tense. Your forehead? Your neck? Your shoulders? This tension inhibits free breathing and makes the body rigid. Your eyes are also feeling this; can you feel the tension around your eyeballs?

c. *The Main Event – PALMING*

Close your eyes now. Do you still feel tension in the eyes? You might be insensitive to the tension because it has been such a chronic part of your life, but if your vision is poor the tension is there. One of your most important challenges is learning how to recognize and relax tension in the eye muscles.

One of the basic methods for relaxing the eye muscles is palming. This method was developed by Dr. Bates, and it can have magical effects on your vision and your general state of relaxation. Palming is so simple that you might at first wonder how it could be of such major help to your vision.

Palming is done by simply cupping your hands over your eyes. Always close your eyes for this exercise. Don't apply any pressure to the eyes themselves, and don't push down on your eyebrows. The purpose is to cover the eyes so that no light gets to them, thus relieving them of any vision "work" and allowing them to relax completely.

Just putting your hands in this position over your eyes should give you an immediate sense of relief from the tension you feel in and around your eyes. Naturally, you will also continue to feel the remaining tension. Don't fight this, simply experience what happens as you palm. Spend a few minutes observing its effects.

It's going to be important for you to find a comfortable position in which to palm, so as to keep tension in your arms and shoulders at a minimum. If you palm while sitting down, make sure you are at a table or desk so that you can prop your elbows up for support. Don't use too low a surface or you'll have to bend your neck and thus cut off the proper flow of circulation to the head and eyes. If you palm lying down, which I find to be the best method, you will probably want to put a pillow or two on your chest for support.

As with all the exercises in this book, don't do too much palming at first. The amount of time you spend doing the exercises is secondary to your frame of mind while doing them. For the first few times, palm for ten nice long easy breaths and then take your hands away. As you palm, allow the blackness to envelop you while you focus on your deep breathing. If thoughts come to mind that take your awareness away from your breathing, gently let those thoughts float off as you bring your attention back to your breathing. It may be some time before your mind will relax for this simple meditation ex-

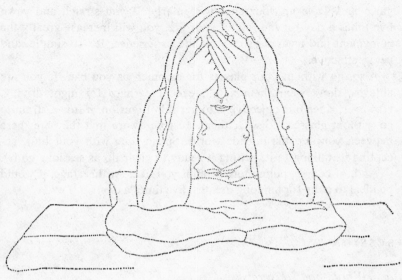

Palming

ercise, and you may find it helpful to count your breaths. In your mind allow the word "one" to rise and then fall with your first breath, and then let "two" effortlessly rise and fall with your second inhalation and exhalation.

When you open your eyes after palming, don't just pop them open and hop up. Wait a bit before opening the eyes, and when you do open them gently, blink a few times and allow a sigh or yawn to come out. And, of course, be aware of how you see. This observation of how you feel after doing an exercise is as important as doing the exercise itself.

IN BETWEEN

In between sessions, you will find that you can do a great deal of exercising while you go about your day. For instance, remember to yawn and wake up your energy regularly. If you stretch and yawn five times a day for the rest of your life, you will increase greatly the enjoyment and awareness of your life experience. It's so simple, and yet so effective.

Also, go without your glasses for as much as you can. If you are able to, don't wear them at all, except perhaps for night driving. However, since our objective is to get rid of tension, if it is a strain to go without glasses, do wear them. Just be aware that they are there between you and the outside world. Spend time with your blur, accepting it, talking to it, getting it ready to clear up as sessions go by.

And, of course, palm more often if you like. At this stage, it would be ideal to palm for ten long breaths, five times a day.

SESSION TWO

a. Whole-body Exercises

This time, while stretching up toward the ceiling, reach up first with one arm and then with the other, rocking your weight from one foot to the other as you do so. Be aware of your spine as you do this, and see if you can feel your vertabrae stretching one by one.

As you stretch, your stomach muscles will relax, and you'll feel a warm flow of energy in the pelvic area. As you reach up with one hand and then the other, allow your hips to have a good stretch so that the rigidity which most of us feel in the lower back and sexual center will have a chance to loosen up. Stretch each side five or six times, breathing deeply and yawning.

Now slowly bring your arms down and bend your body forward at the waist. Keep going forward and down until your fingertips touch the floor in front of you, allowing your knees to bend as much as they need to. Let yourself "hang" as limp and relaxed as a rag doll. Dangle your arms loosely and look back between your legs rather than at the floor, as your head relaxes into the pull of gravity.

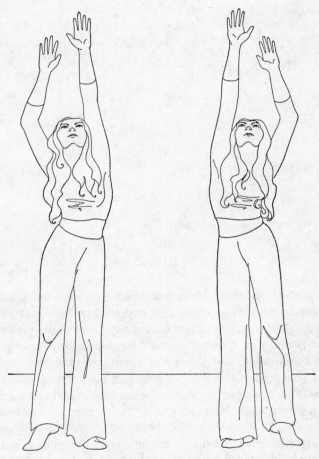

Side Stretching

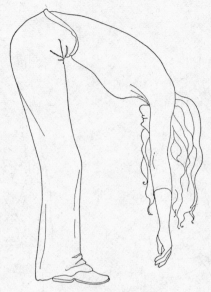

Hanging

As you're "hanging" for a few minutes, notice the sensation of fullness and warmth as blood and oxygen flow into your brain and your eyes. If this feeling at first causes any physical discomfort, stand up slowly and rest. Gradually, you'll be able to stay down longer. If you're comfortable, stay down and breathe deeply. Notice the muscles in your upper lip as they experience the reversal of the pull of gravity. This is happening also to the muscles in and around the eyes.

Flop gently from side to side so that even more of you loosens up. Relax and sigh deeply. Do this about five or six times. When you're ready, slowly straighten up. Keep your arms dangling as you do so, and your chin relaxed on your chest. Stand up from the base of the spine, trying to feel each vertebra come into play as you *gradually* straighten up. Keep breathing easily, and bring your head up last. Stand there quietly with your eyes closed for a moment, focusing on how your body feels, and your eyes in particular. Do this as often in the day as you can, to get maximum benefit.

b.   Eye Warm-ups

With your eyes still closed, tap lightly with your fingertips on the bones surrounding your eyes. You may discover tenderness on the forehead and cheekbones, which comes from tense muscles. The light tapping will help these muscles relax. Breathe deeply as you do this tapping and sigh.

As you open your eyes, allow your eyelids to blink lightly open and shut ten times in a row, with a quick but effortless fluttering. These winks are called "butterfly blinks," and they help bring back the spontaneous blinking habit which tenseness inhibits. Do the series of ten blinks three or four times. In between each series, close the eyes and rest them. If your eyelids tend to snap open and shut instead of blinking effortlessly, be sure to do this exercise several times a day until the movement becomes natural.

Now open your eyes and look into the distance where you find your blur. Let's explore that blur a little further. Consider what would happen if suddenly that blur disappeared and you could see clearly. How would this alter your life, your self-concept, your daily routine? Ask yourself if you really want the blur to clear up—after all, you've spent years perhaps with your blur, you're used to it, you consider it part of you. Even though you would like to see clearly, you may find a certain security in what you are accustomed to, and it can be scary to grow and change and have to face life with a different perspective.

There are certain qualities of that blur which are aesthetically pleasing, at least to me. Notice how your blur gives an impressionistic color panorama to what you see. Many artists strive for this effect in their paintings. Even though your blur keeps you from seeing detail, go ahead and enjoy the color and softened forms you do see.

Remember to blink, breathe, and relax as you look into your blur.

39

Blink—breathe—relax. Remember that normal blinking occurs approximately three times every ten seconds. Good vision is effortless vision. If you "try" to see, you only create tension, and this tension is what is causing you not to see. So give up trying to see into your blur, and just look without trying at all. Does your blur go through changes as you look into it? Be aware of these changes. They are beginning indications that something is happening in your eyes and in your brain, and that "something" is growth!

c. The Main Event—EDGING

In the introductory chapters I discussed the retina and how a small area of the retina, the fovea, is the place where the incoming light is focused for clear vision. Exercises which help you regain your ability to focus light on this area are called centralization exercises, and edging is one of the main centralization exercises.

Edging also helps you overcome your tendency to stare. People with poor vision are habitual starers. If your eyes are frozen in a stare, rather than moving with rapid little movements to see details, your vision doesn't have any chance to see clearly at all. Edging wil help to correct this tendency.

Sit or stand comfortably, and with your eyes pick an object that is just beyond your range of clear vision (without your glasses, of course). Edging is literally looking around the edges of an object, following its outline until you have completely explored it, and then following lines and shapes within the outline of the object, until your brain has been given a complete picture of that object.

Edging is done by moving your entire head. Point your nose in the direction of the object you have chosen and follow the outline of the object, pretending that you are running the tip of your nose along its periphery. This keeps the eyes moving and also keeps them in the proper position for the light to strike the fovea of the retina. As you edge, be sensitive to slight adjustments of your eyes which might bring the object into clearer focus. Little by little, you will find the proper positioning of your head and eyes that gives you the clearest picture.

Go slowly around the edge of the object, feeling any tension and resistance in the eyes, and breathing into that tension to relax it. You will find that at first, your eyes may want to make big jumps rather than make the thousands of tiny movements required to really "take in" an object. Just say to yourself, "slow, slow, slow," to help your eyes relax and do their step-by-step visual process. And remember to blink and breathe as you go along.

Be aware of all the varying degrees of color and shadow as you edge, noticing contrast between background and object. Go around the periphery of the object a few times, and then scan inner details. Remember to keep your head moving and your nose serving as your pointer. Try to relax your neck if it feels tense. Many people with poor vision have tense necks, and this exercise will help relieve that chronic tenseness which inhibits the flow of blood to the head.

Gently memorize what you see, closing your eyes now and then to see if you are retaining an accurate image. Once edging becomes a part of your daily routine, you'll begin to realize just how much you've been missing in your previous way of seeing, with or without glasses. People with poor vision are usually very poor at recalling detail, because they don't edge but stare instead, without really ever looking at an object closely.

Once you have edged enough for your first time, close your eyes and palm for a few moments. In that peaceful blackness, see if you can't visualize the object you edged. Breathe deeply as you experience how your visual memory functions, and don't be upset if it doesn't seem to function very well. We'll be doing many visualization exercises to help your visual memory and imagination recover.

Now let go of the object in your mind's eye and simply relax as you palm. Experience as you palm the "wombian" sensation your eyes might be feeling as you hold your hands protectively over them. Feel the warm peaceful sensation of visually having nothing to do. Rather than palm for ten long breaths as you did in Session One, palm for about five minutes. If you have trouble relaxing, say over and over with each breath, "peaceful, peaceful, peaceful."

IN BETWEEN

Edging is one of the main exercises you can do all the time, so indulge in it throughout your day. Edge the outline of a building, the outline of a person's face and body, the outline of the horizon—edge everything! This is a vital habit to develop if your eyesight is to recover rapidly.

YOUR EYELOGUE

Write down any experiences or insights you had while doing this session's exercises. Enjoy your freedom to put down on paper whatever you want to say.

When you've finished writing about this session, write down how old you were when you got your first pair of glasses. If you can remember, write down the events that led to your going to the optometrist, your experience at the optometrist, and how you felt about your glasses once you got them. Don't bother to go into your emotions at that time, we'll deal with them later. For now, just remember when you got your glasses, and how they felt when you wore them. Go into as much detail as you can remember. This is an important eyelogue entry, and you might want to take an evening or even a week or so to complete it. Don't sit down and feel you have to do it as if it were homework.

Continue with your history of corrective lenses up to the present, writing down how often you got new glasses. How long ago did you get your present pair? How do they feel when you wear them? Put them on and notice the sensation on your nose and ears. If you wear contacts, make notes about what it is like to wear them, as if you were explaining corrective lenses to someone from a culture which didn't have them at all. Write down finally how you feel about wearing corrective lenses.

SESSION THREE

a. *Whole-body Exercises*

For the muscles of the eyes to function properly, they must receive adequate nutrients and be relieved of excess toxins. This means that your circulation must be healthy, your heart must be strong, and your lungs must breathe deeply and regularly. One of the best approaches to healthy circulation is aerobics, a program of physical fitness which gets the heart beating vigorously and the lungs breathing expansively.

The simplest and quickest way to do this right now is to run in place. Just stand up and start running as if you were headed down a quiet secluded country path, but run in place instead of going anywhere. Lift your knees high and really get into the feeling of exerting yourself. Let your breathing become deep and automatic as the requirements of your active body demand more oxygen intake. Stop as soon as you feel yourself laboring to keep going. Then ask yourself these questions:

How long did I run? How did it feel? Did I have to push myself, or was it a positive flow of energy? Does my heart hurt as it thumps away at an accelerated speed or does it feel strong?

These questions are very important to your over-all vision growth from a holistic point of view. It is vital that you find out how fit you are, and then decide what to do if you are not in good physical shape. Refer to the "Suggested Reading" list in the back for books to read for a safe conditioning program.

Regardless of where you are in terms of physical endurance and strength, you can only grow one step at a time. If you jog ten miles a day, great! Just doing that without any specific eye exercises will definitely improve your vision, especially if you jog without your glasses. If, on the other hand, you can't even run in place without fearing your heart will fail you, then you need to find some activity which makes your heart work without pushing you too far. Your heart is a muscle which is sensitive to your emotions and your fears, just as your eyes are. You need to give your heart attention and daily exercise just as you need to give your eyes attention and daily exercise. Eventually you should be able to run in place for fifteen minutes.

For now, be aware of your heart as often as possible, noticing what things you do that make it speed up, and allowing your breathing to go along with that acceleration so that you can develop increased energy and endurance. Also notice how your heartbeat is influenced by your emotions; and how, in turn, the actual functioning of your eyes is affected. To make this association is to make a great step in understanding vision, and in improving your vision through whole-body exercising.

b. Eye Warm-ups

Hopefully you've been edging frequently since the last session. This new exercise uses edging to help you get over the fear of not seeing clearly, and to help you focus on objects. The exercise is called "seeing one thing best," and although it is given here in the warm-up section, it is very important and should be practiced often. You can do this one almost anywhere, anytime, so take advantage of moments throughout the day to "see one thing best."

Sit comfortably with your hands in your lap. Blink and breathe a few moments to relax. Then hold both your thumbs up from your fists, a couple of feet apart so that when you look at one, you see the other in your peripheral vision. You can rest your fists on your thighs or on a table.

First, edge one thumbnail very slowly, breathing deeply and continuing to blink. Remember to use your nose and move your head slightly as you edge the thumbnail. As you are edging, say out loud, "Everything else looks worse." Be aware of your other thumbnail in your peripheral vision. It does indeed look worse, in that it is less clear because you are not looking directly at it.

Now turn your head and look at the other thumbnail and edge it, saying out loud, "Everything else looks worse." Edge slowly and be aware of how clear that thumbnail now is in comparison with the other thumbnail. Go back and forth from one nail to the other, edging each time, and slowly bring the two nails closer together. Even when they are almost touching will they be equally clear in your vision, and even then the one you are edging at the time should seem clearer.

This exercise shows that you do indeed "see one thing best," and that when you want to see something clearly, you must look right at it and let the rest of your peripheral vision be blurry in comparison. People with poor vision tend to either look at the whole field of vision at once without focusing on detail, and to compound the error by turning their heads slightly so that the fovea is not stimulated with the light from the object. Repeat the exercise several times, and palm for several minutes afterward.

c. The Main Event – FUSION

Beginning work with fusion is genuinely main-event action. Fusion refers to the ability of two eyes to look at the same object, to work as a team to bring in a stereoscopic impression of an object which the brain can interpret in three-dimensional images. Many people have fusion trouble, including many people who otherwise have fine vision. If the brain has to strain to interpret images, the result can be a gritty feeling in the eyes, and headaches.

Hold one hand in front of your face, and raise the index finger up while holding the rest of the fingers in a relaxed fist. Look up and down that finger with both eyes and then look beyond the finger at an object in the distance a few feet or more away. What happens? Your eyes shift and focus in the distance, and you find that you are looking between two fingers at the object. This optical illusion gives you a gate through which you can look at the world.

If you continue to get only one finger when you look off into the distance, make sure you're holding your finger directly in front of your face and not off to one side. Stand in front of a mirror if necessary or get a friend to help you get your finger directly in front of

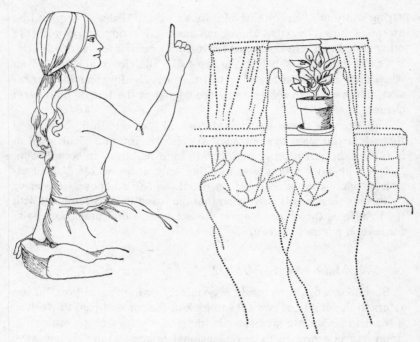

The Finger Gate

your nose. Many people find that one finger is much "stronger" than the other image. This means that one eye, the one opposite the stronger image, is doing most of your seeing, which you can correct.

If you can't get the gate, the object you are looking at in the distance is also a double image, you know that you have definite fusion trouble, and you will need to do special work to correct this problem. Several exercises will be presented in later sessions to regain awareness of your stereoscopic ability, and then you will need to bring those two images together step by step. Don't struggle or "try" to make your eyes get the images together; such effort only creates more tension in the eyes.

Once you have assessed your fusion ability based on this test, carry the exercise a step further by moving your finger and your head from side to side as you look through your "gate." Slowly move the finger to the left, then to the right, keeping your head moving along with the finger. Take your time; breathe, blink! Find an object that is fairly large, and edge it as you swing your gate back and forth. Swing and edge through your finger for two or three minutes.

With this exercise you are helping your eyes to learn to "let go" of separate images, to move quickly from one fixation to another without holding on to a particular image. This tendency to "hold on" to an image rather than edging and taking on many rapid pictures of an object is characteristic of people with poor vision. There is a general personality trait of being afraid to "let go," to be in motion, to risk giving up one thing in order to open up to other things and a greater vision of life. This fear can be greatly reduced through these simple exercises, so that as you look through your gate and force your eyes to move and not hold on, you're also helping your general personality to loosen up and realize that there is nothing to fear in letting go.

IN BETWEEN

Develop a physical-fitness program which suits your needs. Genuine aerobics requires that you run long enough, or swim or jump rope, etc. long enough and vigorously enough, to where your heart definitely gets a rigorous workout. Aim toward this goal, but don't overdo and try for a sudden change in your physical condition.

For the rest of your life you will want to be aware that you are seeing "one thing best," so make this a conscious habit. The finger gate is so simple to do at any time and wherever you are; combine it with edging so that your clear spot of vision scans your environment without staring at one small spot.

Begin to gain confidence that you are on the right path. Change takes time, and since your eyes are an integral part of your whole being, you must be aware that your whole being is changing for the better as you face your dangers, begin to open up visually and emotionally, and gain a clearer picture of reality.

Visionetics

Of course, looking at your world you won't automatically make everything out there okay. The Russians still have their missiles pointed at us, we're still running out of energy, and we're always having to deal with interpersonal relationships and economic risks. But we can choose how we will respond to these threats. Instead of reacting with fear and tension, with anxiety and withdrawal, we can accept the dangers inherent in life, get over childhood panic reactions, and live openly and consciously. It is the chronic unconscious anxiety which is the real problem to vision and tension. It is the ingrained habit which hinders vision to such an extent that we can't consciously see clearly. So through these exercises you will be overcoming habitual tension so that you can deal directly and openly with the present world out there, with vision that is clear enough to give you a good chance of dealing with whatever you encounter.

SESSION FOUR

a.   *Whole-body Exercises*

This yoga exercise is called "the chest expander." It will relieve shoulder tension, increase your circulation, and also your air intake, so breathe gently while you're still learning it, so that you don't become dizzy. Stand comfortably and well balanced, with your feet six inches to a foot apart. Stretch both arms out to the sides at shoulder height. Take a deep breath and bring your arms straight out in front of you with a slow graceful gesture. Place the fingertips together with palms facing away, and continue to breathe deeply as you slowly bring your arms around each side to touch behind your back.

Clasp your hands together behind your back and, keeping them clasped, slowly raise them as high as you comfortably can toward the ceiling or sky. At the same time, tuck your hips under and stretch up to the ceiling with your whole body, inhaling deeply through your nose. Hold the stretch for as long as it feels invigorating.

Now, as you exhale, keep your hands high and still clasped in back

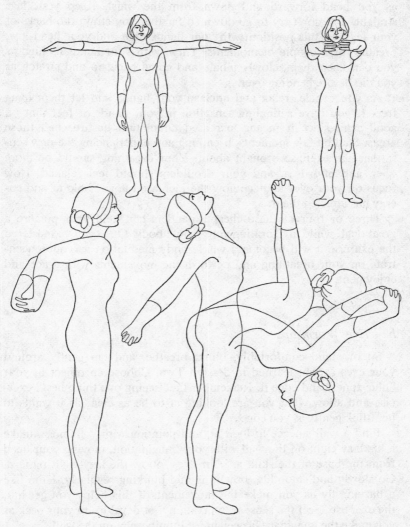

The Chest Expander

as you bend forward and down from the waist. Keep your legs straight, and don't try to go down so far that you strain the backs of your legs. In this position with your hands high and your head low, breathe for a couple of moments. Then, with your hands as high as you can keep them, slowly inhale and come back up and stretch as you did before bending over.

As you exhale, relax and unclasp your hands and let them hang free. If you have a tingling sensation in your hands or feet that's a good sign, since it means increased circulation has reached those areas. Stand a few moments, breathing and experiencing the new sensations the exercise brought about. Your breathing should be more open and effortless, and your shoulders should feel relaxed. Now focus on your eyes and see how the increased flow of blood and energy has affected them.

Three or four of these chest expanders can help your posture a great deal, while invigorating your whole body. Once you've mastered the exercise it will become a whole-body meditation as you concentrate on your breathing and perform the movements with grace and enjoyment.

b. Eye Warm-ups

Sit or stand comfortably, blink, breathe, and tap gently around your eyes as you learned in Session Two. Choose an object in your "blur zone," and edge it. Remember the "seeing one thing best" exercise and allow what you are looking at to be as clear as it wants to be. Blink gently as you edge.

Find a wall surface to look at, and pointing with your nose, make a big lazy eight on the wall with your imagination, moving your head from the base of the skull as your eyes follow the lazy-eight pattern. Go slowly and smoothly, breathing and blinking regularly. Hum like a buzzing fly as you make the movements if this helps you get into the exercise. Feel the sense of relaxation that develops in your neck as you make the imaginary lazy eight, or infinity sign, on the wall.

Do your eyes seem to jerk from one place on the lazy eight to another, leaving big gaps in the curves? This exercise is designed to help the eyes regain their natural vibratory movement as they rapidly shift along the curved line of the lazy eight. Your eyes should be firing off hundreds of rapid images to your brain as you do a lazy eight, in order for you to be seeing well.

c. The Main Event – SHORT SWINGS

Swings are perhaps the most effective way to get the eyes shifting in their natural vibratory pattern. There are long swings and short swings, swings done with the eyes open (such as the lazy-eight swing you just did), and swings done with the eyes closed. As with so many of the Bates exercises, from which these are derived, swings are so simple that people often don't believe they can actually help bring about vision recovery. Don't be deceived by this simplicity; the longer and more often you swing, the better. You can't possibly do too much swinging, and the sooner you turn the exercises into enjoyable meditations the quicker your brain will integrate the experience into growth and relaxation.

We'll do one short swing in this session, and then in later sessions I'll introduce more for variety. These exercises should be done with a sense of playfulness rather than with sober determination, so relax and enjoy yourself!

The "painting swings" we'll do in this session should be done with your eyes closed, but before you do so, look around the room. Let your eyes take in the most outstanding colors and objects, and then close your eyes and visualize the scene in your mind's eye.

Now imagine that you have a long weightless telescoping paint-brush attached to the end of your nose. You're going to "paint" over the room you just looked at. Choose any color to start with, red or blue for instance, and begin painting with bold, broad strokes. Start close to your chair and gently sweep your head back and forth with your eyes closed as the brush leaves pure solid color everywhere you point it.

Gradually allow your strokes to expand and see the paint covering

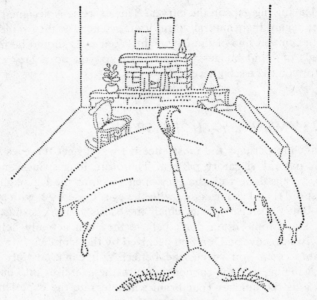

The Painting Swing

more and more of the furniture, the walls, the floor, with a beautiful solid color. Color the whole room or environment, and then choose another color and start painting over the old color. Have fun! Use as many colors and coats of paint as you have the concentration and time for, but do paint the room at least four different colors. Breathe with each stroke of the brush so that you establish a rhythmic pattern of painting and breathing. Sigh as often as you wish, to keep your swings flowing and relaxed.

Don't worry if you cannot vividly picture all of this in your mind; people with poor vision often have difficulty visualizing. If your mind comes up with a complete blank while you pretend to paint, go ahead and act out the painting anyway, enjoying the sensation in your neck and head as you swing back and forth. As with the other visual abilities, you can't "make" yourself visualize—you must simply do exercises which encourage the visualization process to come alive again.

As you are swinging, your eyes will be closed and relaxed, but your head will be in motion and your mind will be looking at what you are imagining. This motion and inner looking will encourage your eyes to shift with freedom, to scan and edge without having to deal with the outside world. Such a relaxed visual experience can do wonders for your eyes, as you will find when you open your eyes after a few minutes or perhaps even ten minutes of "painting swings."

When you do open your eyes, look around the room while you blink, breathe, and relax. How do you see the room now? If you see better, excellent! These exercises may sometimes give you flashes of clearer vision which will grow in duration and clarity as you continue to do the exercises. But, of course, don't get discouraged if you feel your eyesight isn't improving in leaps and bounds. If you focus instead on enjoying your sessions and in becoming more centered, energized, and relaxed, your eyes will naturally improve.

IN BETWEEN

Take this painting swing and have fun with it. Whenever you have even just a moment, close your eyes and paint your environment with your favorite color. Remember not to get into detailed painting, which will inhibit the free swinging of your head, just have fun slopping around the paint.

For variation, paint your lazy-eight, or infinity symbol, on walls. Or your initials, or whatever you want to paint. Let your imagination do whatever it desires to do. This will directly loosen up your visual ability.

As with all the exercises, you might find that doing this painting swing around friends makes you feel embarrassed. Be open about the fact that you're following a program on vision improvement and that what you are doing is simply an exercise. Since over 50 per cent of your friends probably need to do the exercises themselves, you might find that a small group of you will start doing the exercises together.

YOUR EYELOGUE

Write down any frustrations you had with this session's exercises and also any flashes of clarity or insights. Did you have fun? Did you learn anything about your ability to visualize?

In your eyelogue entry last session you began exploring when you first got glasses, and how your glasses currently feel when you wear them. For this session, here is a sentence-completion exercise to further explore your relationship with your corrective lenses. I'll give you the beginning of a sentence, and you complete it however you wish. Write different endings to explore the different ramifications of the sentence. Just write whatever comes to mind; don't pause and reflect. This exercise is designed to bring out how you *feel* about wearing corrective lenses, not how you *think* about wearing them. So just write anything, even if the first couple of sentences come out as nonsense. Here's the beginning for you:

"If I never wore my corrective lenses (glasses or contacts) again . . . ."

SESSION FIVE

a. Whole-body Exercises

The following exercise is drawn from the yogic tradition and is usually called the "sponge" because during the exercise you soak up relaxation while you rest on your back on the floor. When you master this exercise you will be able to lie quietly in a state of complete physical and mental relaxation, and your whole body, including your eyes, will benefit greatly. (This exercise is excellent for helping you relax into sleep at night, but it is also an energizing exercise for other parts of the day.)

Find a quiet, secure place where you can spend twenty minutes without interruption. Loosen or remove any constricting clothing and lie down on your back on a firm, but padded surface. Take a few deep breaths, and make sure that your body is straight. Raise your head to check by looking down at your legs, and make any necessary adjustments. It's amazing how often we feel we're aligned when, in fact, our body is crooked.

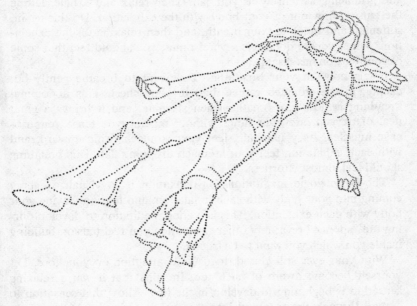

The Sponge

Rest with your feet comfortably apart and your arms relaxed at your side. Let your feet flop apart and your palms face the ceiling. If your lower back hurts you in this position, bend your knees and tuck your hips to flatten your back against the floor. After a few minutes with your back flattened against the floor lower your knees again and see if the pain has been relieved. If not, do this exercise with your knees bent. You won't be able to relax if your back is hurting you.

Now close your eyes and focus your awareness on how your body feels. Make note of the tenseness you may feel in different parts of your body. Before moving into deep relaxation, let's relieve some of that tension through counter-tension release. Make fists of your hands and stiffen your whole body for a moment, holding your breath and grimacing as tensely as you can. Then relax and exhale, letting the tension flow out of your body with the exhalation. Do this again, stiffening and inhaling your breath, and then relaxing on the exhalation. When you've done this several times, you should feel that some of your tension has disappeared.

Focus now on your breathing. You want to breathe gently but deeply, in the stomach rather than in your chest. This abdominal breathing is how you breathe when sleeping, and it brings a great deal of oxygen into your lungs without making you tense your ribcage muscles. As you inhale, feel your stomach rising upward, and with each exhalation feel your stomach dropping flat. This breathing should feel almost effortless.

The basic yogic meditation for relaxation is to visualize energy coming into your body with each inhalation, and tension leaving your body with each exhalation. This is a good meditation to develop during the "sponge" or at any other time when you feel tension building inside you which you want to be free of.

With your eyes still closed, focus your attention on your toes. Let yourself become aware of each toe. Imagine that a warm relaxing sensation is beginning to develop in the tips. Allow that sensation to spread through the toes and into the arches and soles of your feet. Move your feet a little to feel that they are beginning to give into the warm relaxing sensation and go limp, free of tension.

Allow this warm sensation of relaxation to flow up into your ankles, and then on up into your calf muscles. If you feel resistance to the flow of relaxation, tense the resisting muscles and then relax them, as you did your whole body earlier. Stay in tune with your breathing, exhaling that tension and inhaling the sensation of relaxation with each breath.

Allow the warm relaxation to flow up into your knees.

Concentrate on your thighs and let go of the tension there. Let the muscles relax layer by layer until you feel you are melting into the floor.

Imagine that your hip joints are loose and open and flexible, and that the relaxation is flowing into your sexual parts with a warm relaxed good feeling. Rock your pelvis a couple of times to feel this sensation of well-being and to be sure that your muscles in that area are all relaxing and giving in to the sensation of peace and pleasurable calmness.

Now let that relaxed flow move on into your stomach and lower back. Feel your breathing being suffused with light, pleasurable sensations. Let the tension drain away as you begin to feel almost weightless. Your internal organs are relaxing as well—allow that relaxation to move up your spine and eliminate the tension of the muscles on either side of your spinal cord.

Your rib cage is rising and falling slightly.

Your heart is beating without effort or tension, doing its work but not straining.

Your lungs are taking in energy, expelling tension.

Let your shoulders relax as your chest opens up to the relaxed sensation of security and lightness.

Shift your awareness to your fingertips, where the warm sensation of relaxation is beginning to grow. Become aware of each of your fingers as the blood circulates with a warm pulsing of relaxation and well-being. Your hands may feel very light as the relaxation fills them and the draining tension leaves them. Allow this sensation to flow up your arms, dispelling the tension in the muscles all the way up to the shoulders. Your shoulder muscles relax even more, and you feel your entire body giving in to the pull of gravity and melting peacefully into the floor.

Focus on your neck and throat muscles. Exhale with a barely audible sigh and let the tension in your vocal cords relax and disappear.

Relax your jaw. Move it around a little to help the tension disappear if you want to. Let your jaw hang limp and free of tension. Also, allow the sensation of warm relaxation to free your tongue of constriction.

Your lips also; let them relax as you sigh again.

Your cheek muscles relax, and the area where your head is touching the floor relaxes. Your scalp relaxes. Perhaps you want to make a squinting face to get in touch with your forehead and eyes. Tense them and then relax and let the tension disappear. The relaxation in your whole body flows upward and fills your head, bringing a fluttering sense of release to your eyes as the tension fades away and a profound sense of peace and quiet fills your eyes. This sensation of relaxation is now glowing throughout your body, mind, and spirit as your breathing fills your consciousness and relaxes your mind of any thoughts or concerns. You are completely relaxed, at peace, content.

Effortlessly you remain with your entire being relaxed as you just rest and breathe in energy and well-being.

You may stay in this relaxed state for as long as you wish. When you are ready to rise, your breathing will accelerate, your eyes will open, and a great yawn and stretch will run from one end of your body to the other as the energy flows freely through you. With your eyes open and your body at rest, allow the light to enter your eyes and your brain as if the light were more relaxation and energy. Let the light shine in without doing anything about it. Just experience your sense of vision when it is free of any care or tension. Stay with this feeling as you slowly sit up and end the exercise.

What you just did with your whole body is what you are wanting to do with your eye muscles in particular. As your brain learns to focus on a calf muscle or a finger, it can learn to focus on an extraocular eye muscle so that relaxation can occur there where it is most needed.

b. *Eye Warm-ups*

In this exercise we'll be working on accommodation, which is the shifting of the eyes' focus from near to far, and vice versa. As mentioned in the introductory chapters, scientists are still arguing about how this shifting of focus takes place, disagreeing as to whether the lens does the shifting or the muscles surrounding the eyes do the shifting by altering the shape of the eyeball itself. Regardless of what side one takes in this argument (I personally feel both factors come into play in accommodation), the inability to make this shift is a major cause in either near- or farsightedness, and such exercises as "whipping" will begin to increase your accommodation ability.

This exercise gives the eye muscles a good workout, so we will follow it with palming. This pattern of doing an exercise and then palming is basic to most of the exercises we'll be doing. When doing the sponge, I suggested that you tense your muscles first, and then relax after that extreme tension. This is also what happens when you whip and then palm. One of the major drawbacks of standard optometric eye exercises is that twenty minutes of exercising (tensing) are usually terminated without the vital healing effects of palming immediately following.

Whipping is an exercise which presbyopes (farsighted people) and high myopes (very nearsighted people) will want to do with great regularity. You might not notice visual improvement at first, but stay with it because it gets right at those spasmed muscles, which have been behind corrective lenses for some time, and which may be somewhat slow to respond.

Decide if you have a weaker eye and a stronger eye, or if your eyes are basically the same. If one eye is worse than the other, it will need a lot of whipping in the next few weeks, followed of course by palming each time. But work with the other eye also.

To begin, cup your right hand over your left eye, but keep both eyes open so they blink and move together. This crossing over with the arm is important so that the eye doesn't get pulled out of alignment. You'll be whipping with your left hand and your right eye first. Hold your left hand out as far to the left as you can while still keeping it in sight of the right eye. Keep watching your left palm as you bring it in toward the right eye with a moderately rapid movement. Bring the hand to within a few inches of the eye and then whip it back out to the extreme position with moderate speed. Watch a particular line in your palm so the eye has something to focus on. Even

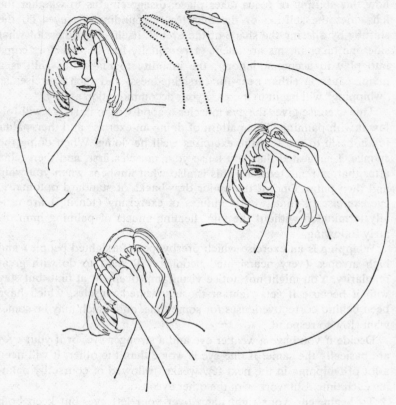

Whipping

if the line doesn't stay clear as you whip in and out, your eye will still be changing its focus. This, as you can feel in your eye, is quite strenuous work for those accommodation muscles, so remember to stay relaxed by breathing regularly and deeply, and blinking often. Once you have done this whipping in and out ten or twelve times, change eyes and hands and whip on the other side. Stay with the exercise for several minutes, until your concentration begins to fade, and then palm until any feeling of strain is gone.

I can't overemphasize the importance of this exercise. It is particularly helpful for presbyopes who are supposed to have dying inelastic lenses. When the exercise is new it might feel like a strain, but once you get into it you will enjoy the exercise, and you'll be able to do it for longer and longer periods of time. You should work up to five minutes at a time on each eye.

c. The Main Event – FINGER-SHIFT FUSION

We'll continue teaching the eyes to work together with the following finger-shift fusion exercise. Hold up your index fingers in front of your face, one about six inches from your nose and the other finger a foot or so farther out. First look at the finger closest to you. What happens? You see two fingers beyond that first finger: one on each side of it.

Now shift your focus to the farther finger. The first finger will now appear to have become two fingers. Shift back and forth five or six times and be aware of how this feels to your eyes. Then, look into the distance past both fingers, and both will appear as double images, or two gates. Now do five sets of shifting: from the first finger to the second, and then out again into the distance. Then palm until your eyes feel renewed.

Now focus on the first finger again, and while holding your gaze there, drop the finger down; you should retain the image of two fingers in the background. Hold that image for about a minute if you can. Do this exercise for about five minutes per day of trying to hold the phantom image.

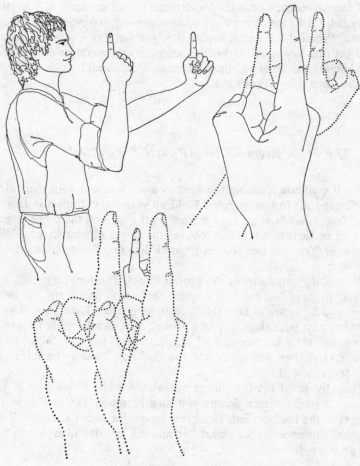

The Finger Shift

YOUR EYELOGUE

We are now a quarter of the way through this program, and it would be a good idea for you to write down your feelings thus far about the program itself, how you have been responding to it, and whether or not you've integrated the first five sessions adequately and are ready to go on.

Also, make note of how you feel about looking into your "blur zone" now that you've been doing some exercises designed to penetrate that zone with clear vision. How does your blur look these days? Any clearer?

How do you feel about seeing in general these days? Are you enjoying looking at things more, are you letting your outside world come inside you with less resistance?

Once you have finished with your eyelogue, remember to palm! Whenever you read or do other somewhat straining work with your eyes, palm for a few moments or minutes. This is so important I can't stress it enough. Also, stay aware of when you wear your glasses or contacts, and notice the times you keep them on or in when you don't need them to get by. Contacts are insidious in that they're so hard to take in and out. You might consider wearing your glasses more and your contacts less, especially if you have an old pair of glasses with a weaker prescription than your contacts. This would give you more freedom in taking off your glasses when you don't really need them.

I should point out that I'm not really an enemy of glasses. They have their place, and they do give you a clarity of vision which is interesting aesthetically as well as practically. Remember that 20/20 isn't any absolute. Vision is a sense for perceiving the environment in a pleasing, aesthetic, and practically efficient way. And as you already know, my bias is that the natural way is holistically the "best" way. Glasses aren't evil, they simply inhibit the natural functioning of the body's visual organs.

SESSION SIX

a. *Whole-body Exercises*

In his excellent book *Bioenergetics,* Alexander Lowen mentions that if we could only massage the muscles surrounding the eyes as we massage other muscles of the body, visual tension could be decreased very rapidly. Unfortunately, most of the muscles surrounding the eyes cannot be reached from the outside, so physical manipulation is impossible. However, there are a number of massage techniques which can directly help the eyes, and we will be doing one of these in this session.

Massage, whether self-administered or shared with another person, is one of the finest aids to holistic health, both at the physical and the mental level of relaxation. The laying on of hands not only increases circulation and promotes muscular relaxation, it is also a direct expression of love and concern. The wake-up massage we will be doing in this session is self-massage, letting your eyes know first thing in the morning that you want to help them.

This four-step massage can be done any time during the day, but it is most beneficial right after you awaken in the morning.

Before starting the massage, lie on your back and indulge in a few good stretches and yawns and general wiggles of your body to start your circulation flowing and your breathing going more vigorously.

The first step of the massage, done with your eyes closed, is a gentle pounding around the bony perimeter of the eyes with your middle fingers. Use just the first joint of the fingers for best results. Start on the upper inside part of the bony ridge above your eyes, and go all the way around and then back again the other way. Do this perhaps ten times, using quick firm beating movements. This might be a sensitive area for you and could hurt a little as you pound. Don't beat so hard as to cause real pain, but do stimulate those tender areas. As

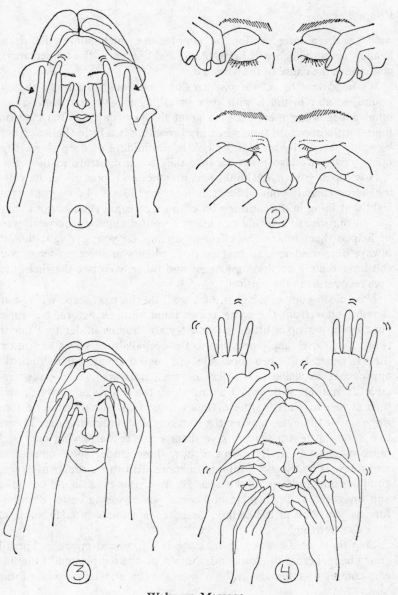

Wake-up Massage

we'll see in a later session on acupressure, such stimulation is a healing action which will bring blood and energy to the tender areas and relieve the cause of the soreness.

It's important to get the oxygen flowing through the body as you pound, so stay in touch with your breathing to give your awakening mind a beginning meditation to greet the new day. I often sing or hum a little nonsense tune when my breathing is a little shallow from being awakened by an alarm clock in the middle of deep sleep. Big noisy yawns are also great because they bring moisture to the eyes.

Now open your eyes, blink, and breathe, and look up at the ceiling. How clear is your vision this morning? Get to know your eyesight first thing in the morning based on a constant such as your ceiling, so that right away you can know if your dreams tensed your eyes or helped them relax. The effect of dreams on your eyesight should always be considered, so that on days when you wake up tense you can immediately do these massages and other exercises that help the eyes recover from the tension.

Now close your eyes again, and we'll do the next step. With your thumbs, start from the same upper inner spot as before, but raise your eyebrows up a little and insert your thumbs under that upper ridge. Don't ever apply pressure to the eyeballs themselves as you do this (in general, this is a good rule, although there are some "radical" approaches to vision aid which use such pressure). Just make tiny circular motions with your thumbs along the top ridge outward, and then switch to your middle or index fingers to go along the bottom ridge under the eyes, making the same small circular motions. If certain spots are extra tender, give them extra tender loving care and more massage time. Be aware of how these tender spots change as mornings go by. Spend a minute or more with this circular massage, going around and around the eyes. By now your eyes should be moist and invigorated. Open them and see if you're seeing better than before as you look at the ceiling. Breathe, remember to edge, and get your eyes moving!

Step three of the wake-up massage is a forehead massage. Spread your fingers across the forehead, thumbs on the temples and little fingers coming together above the nose in the center. The purpose of this exercise is to rub the fingers, one hand at a time, upward to the hairline. Do not stroke downward, but up again with quick firm movements vigorously over the skin, left to right, left to right, left to right. Don't press too hard. People with poor eyesight often have a chronic frown or squint, and these muscles need to be pushed in the opposite direction regularly to relax them and remind them that they don't have to tense downward over the eyes. Your forehead should feel warm, loose, and invigorated when you've done this for a minute or longer. Breathe deeply, hum or yawn with abandon, and don't rub yourself raw through too much enthusiasm.

The final step of this wake-up massage is a finishing touch which gets rid of the remaining tension and poor circulation. Lightly run your fingers from your chin up to the top of your head and then fling off the accumulated tension into the atmosphere with a flick of your fingers. There is much controversy about the actual presence of such negative energy which can be picked up by running hands over the surface of one's body. Scientifically no one can say what is happening when you do this, but you will feel a definite sensation that does indeed help relax your face and eyes, and if it works for you it doesn't matter if it can be explained scientifically; do it because it feels good and let your experience be your judge of its validity.

Don't run your fingers directly over the eyes as you do this, just lightly touch your face with ten or fifteen little dashes upward. Your face should feel tingly and alive when you're finished. I've found that many people are so invigorated by this four-part massage that they give up their morning cigarette or cup of coffee because they like the way they feel naturally. Give it a try for a few weeks, and see if you don't pick up this healthy habit as the best way to start your new day.

Also, do this massage any time during the day when you feel tension building up in your eyes and face. Such self-help can greatly change your life for the better. It's yet another of those little things which make a big difference in your day.

b. Eye Warm-ups

Sit comfortably and look around you. As you look, see how many bad habits you can catch yourself doing, and use the exercises you've learned to correct those bad habits. How does your vision respond? How are your eyes feeling in general today? How tense do they feel? Do they want to see what is out there, or is there an inner resistance?

Palm for a couple of minutes, breathing deeply and meditating on your breathing and on relaxing into the warm blackness of the visual field behind your closed eyes and palms.

Now open your eyes and look around you again. Blink, breathe, edge, relax, see! How is your blur doing now?

Close your eyes again and palm another few minutes, and this time say to yourself, "What's out there that I'm afraid to see?" Meditate on this question and see what answers pop into your mind, regardless of their validity. Simply begin to explore your possible apprehensions. Probably you will find that you no longer have anything to fear but fear itself, and facing that fear will show it for what it is—nothing but a blur.

Now open your eyes, saying to yourself, "I'm not afraid of what's out there." Say this several times as a positive affirmation, and see how your vision responds to this positive thought.

c. The Main Event – THE NEAR-FAR CHART

We're now going to do one of the more powerful exercises for bringing your blur into clear focus. I call this exercise the near-far chart exercise. It is an accommodation exercise which works directly on your ability to change your focus from near to far, or vice versa if you're presbyopic (farsighted).

You will find the near-far chart below. Make a duplicate of this chart on an index card. Put the chart with the large letters up on your wall considerably into your "blur zone" but not so far away it is a total blur. If you are farsighted this large-letter chart will be clear to you, of course, and you will do the exercise in reverse of myopes (nearsighted people). Now sit comfortably with the small-letter chart in your hand where you can make out the letters. The exercise consists of looking at the first letter on the chart that you can see clearly, and then looking quickly at the other chart at the same first letter which is blurry. Don't bother "trying" to see the blurry letter clearly, just look where it is, and quickly look back at the second letter on your clear chart, and back at the second letter on the blurry chart. Continue to do this with the rest of the letters until your concentration fades or your eyes feel strained. You should be able to work up to fifteen minutes on the chart. Remember to blink and breathe!

When your eyes feel they have had enough, immediately palm for a few minutes. While you palm, either meditate on the warm black safety you are experiencing visually, or visualize the blurry chart in your mind's eye and see if it won't become clear in your imagination. If not, visualize the clear chart first and then look at the blurry chart and see if you can't imagine it clearing up. Breathe deeply, and don't be frustrated if the first few times you do this exercise you can't clear up the blurry chart. Be patient.

After you have palmed awhile, open your eyes, blink and look at the blurry chart, and see if you don't see it more clearly than you did before.

Now repeat the near-far chart exercise, taking your time, and being sure not to tense and "try to see." The purpose of this exercise is to get those eye muscles to relax and do their work, not to tense under a mental strain of trying to succeed.

When you've done the near-far exercise enough, palm again. See if you can visualize the blurry chart and allow it to become as clear as your clear chart. Then just relax and as you palm, say to yourself, "I can see clearly," over and over again. When you open your eyes, look at the chart and see if your desire is beginning to come true, but don't lay expectations on your eyes, just continue to open up to seeing into your blur.

```
F 8 Y U 4
3 K Z L P
N Q E M I
C Y P B 4
X C R 9 T
O 3 J V W
7 X 5 2 S
A W I R C
J R N 2 D
B 3 Z W I
```

```
W  H  T  M  5
S  2  G  B  A
R  7  X  C  9
6  O  J  L  3
L  G  K  6  N
E  Y  U  F  D
8  Q  O  G  T
P  L  M  B  3
Y  F  E  8  V
9  T  R  6  Q
```

IN BETWEEN

You can do many variations on the near-far chart exercise throughout the day. For instance, at work or wherever, you can look at your watch every fifteen minutes and then look in the distance at the same number on a clock which has big letters but is farther away. Also, you can get a small calendar for your desk and a large calendar for the wall, and each day look from the date that is blurry to the date that is clear, and in doing this you will help your eyes greatly.

SESSION SEVEN

a. *Whole-body Exercises*

Go through the stretching and yawning exercise, and then flop over loosely as you learned in Session Two. Follow this with the chest expander, remembering to focus on your breathing. This quick whole-body warm-up takes only a few minutes, so make it a regular habit if you enjoy it.

Now let's do some upper-body and hip rotations to further extend the stretching routine and loosen up more of the body. These rotations are especially designed to energize the pelvic area and to free the tension that gets blocked in the sexual area so that you have a more complete flow of energy throughout your body.

Assume a comfortable stance, with clothes loosened or removed. Place your hands on your hips, with your feet a foot or so apart. Turn your toes in slightly, and bend forward at the waist as you begin to rotate the top half of your body in wide circles. Start with little circles if you're feeling stiff, and slowly make wider ones as you loosen up. Go around to the right three or four times, and then reverse the direction. Breathe and blink!

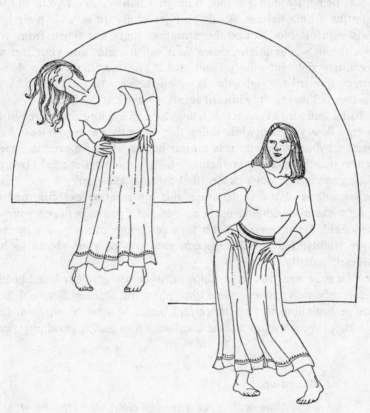

Upper-body and Hip Rotations

Next rotate just the hips themselves, to loosen up the pelvic area. This crucial point of energy blockage may seem a long way from the eyes, but if there is chronic tension in the pelvis it will affect the whole being, including vision. With your hands still on your hips, rotate like a hula dancer, slowly and gracefully, in as wide a circle as feels comfortable. Notice the sensation that runs down from your hips through your thighs, down your calf muscles into your feet and seemingly right into the ground. See if you can't also feel a flow of energy upward through your body all the way to your head; having the toes pointed slightly inward seems to augment this feeling.

More and more research is being done to explore the source of the energy flow you feel while doing this and other energy-release exercises. Obviously, gravity acts on our bodies while we exercise, and it is also possible that we are actually feeling the magnetic field that our body generates through its electrochemical nerve-energy flow.

Regardless of the explanation, this hip rotation exercise, and the energy exercises coming up later, will help you experience your energy field. Being aware of this flow of energy can not only increase your vitality, but it will also convince you of your ability to heal yourself visually.

You may want to run in place or otherwise get your heart beating vigorously now, to complete this phase of Session Seven. I hope you're beginning to feel better and better in your body, or at least working through tensions that keep you from feeling good physically.

b. *Eye Warm-ups*

Spend some time with your near-far chart. You might want to begin keeping close track of how your vision varies day by day, or even minute by minute. If you have your large-letter chart permanently on a wall, stand or sit in front of it right where the letters begin to blur. Mark this spot by leaving a chair there, and measure how many feet and inches you are from the chart when the letters begin to lose their clarity. Make a note of this in your eyelogue for future reference as you'll want to gauge your progress as you move from the chart.

At about a foot beyond your clear-vision distance, stand or sit and look at the letters while you breathe deeply and blink. Without making an effort, you might find the letters clearing up for you. Palm for a minute or two, breathing deeply and relaxing your eyes. Think the word "clear" as a mantra if you like while you palm. Then open your eyes, blink gently, and look at the chart. Did it clear up more?

Now do some whipping exercises with the palm of your hand. Then palm. Then look at the chart and see if it has cleared up even more for you. Begin to accept that your eyesight is a sensitive variable of your whole personality, and that it changes all the time. We are conditioned to believe that there is one "proper" way to see things, but in actuality every time we look at something, we see it in a unique way because we are changing, growing organisms, not static visual machines. The tendency of myopes to hold on to something, to want things to stay the same, is a defensive action which thwarts the natural fluid flexibility of healthy vision, and the more you accept that the world is a constantly changing, alive, growing process the more your vision will relax, take on this responsive quality, and become the amazing sense organ which it is potentially.

To finish up this session's warm-ups, do some short swings with your eyes closed, painting the room with your nose paintbrush. If you want some variation on that theme, do the "picket fence" short swing. Imagine a white picket fence across a street from you. You have a telescoping stick attached to your nose, and as you rotate your head from the base of your skull back and forth from side to side, you run your stick along the fence. The stick hits each one of the pickets in rapid succession, and your eyes follow the movement of the nose and look at each picket board as it is hit. This gets the eyes shifting very well. Imagine you can hear the clicking of your stick on the picket fence as you move along it.

If you're nearsighted, imagine the fence getting farther and farther away while you continue to see the individual pickets clearly. Reverse this if your eyes are farsighted. Breathe! And enjoy your game as if you were Huckleberry Finn without a care in the world right at that moment. This exercise will increase eye shifting as well as your ability to visualize clearly.

c. The Main Event – LONG SWINGS

We're now going to take short swinging and expand it to include the whole body, rather than just the head and neck. The long swings should not replace short swings, although they are extremely powerful and can bring about rapid visual improvement. Long swings are usually done with the eyes open (compared to short swings, usually done with the eyes closed), and they are done standing up. Do them outside in the sunlight if you can.

Stand so that you have a good sense of balance, but don't place your feet too far apart. Allow your hands to hang loosely, keep your head level, and begin to gently swing back and forth. As you swing back and forth you will be shifting your weight from one foot to the other, but not raising your feet off the ground. Your heel will come off the ground in a golfer's swing, so that as you swing to the right, your left heel rises a little as your weight goes on the right foot, and vice versa.

Keep your torso fairly still so that the swinging takes place in your hips rather than higher in your waist. Don't swing so fast that your arms fly away from your body. This is a gentle whole-body swing into which you breathe and relax.

Your head should follow your body as it swings. Don't look at anything in particular, just let your eyes slide past the horizontal view while you keep an attitude of relaxed curiosity. Your interest is in watching the world go by, not in holding on to any particular object. The more you do this swing, the more you will begin to experience the optical illusion that the outside world is sliding past you in the opposite direction. When this starts to happen, your long swings are be-

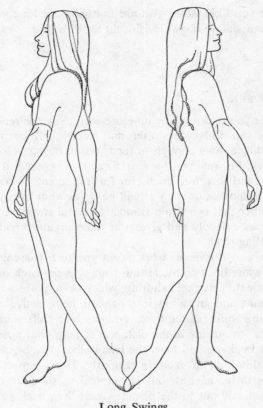

Long Swings

ginning to work their magic. You have let go, your eye muscles are relaxed and not "trying" to see anything, and the natural optical illusion which should happen is happening.

If at first the swinging makes you dizzy, ease off and do it very gently and for a shorter time, but do it every day until the dizziness or nausea disappears, and you find yourself enjoying the sensation of floating free as the world goes by. Swing for at least two minutes and

77

up to ten if you like. When you are finished with long swings, sit or lie down and palm. If you wish, check with your eye chart after palming.

IN BETWEEN

Whenever you're doing any up-close work, such as reading or sewing, etc., be sure to look up often and shift your focus momentarily into the distance, long enough to focus on an object before returning to your work. For myopes, look up first at an object just within your clear range, and then into your blur for a moment. If you then palm every fifteen minutes or so, you will be doing your eyes a great service. Remember that eye strain is mostly mental strain while using the eyes, so breathe deeply and give your mind regular breaks from tension-generating work.

You can also do vision work when you're a passenger in a car. Watch the white lines go by, letting your eyes see each one, and then shift to the next. This rapid shifting, which takes place so quickly that you must relax and just allow it to happen, helps activate the spontaneous shifting ability of the eyes. You can also shift your focus from inside the car to outside in the distance, to help your accommodation muscles get in shape and keep the lens limber. Presbyopes especially should do this kind of exercise regularly. Don't expect the shift in focus to be instantaneous, but rather feel as though your vision is sliding effortlessly out to the distance, and then back to near vision.

YOUR EYELOGUE

For this session, I'd like you to begin thinking about the emotional climate you were living in when you became aware that your eyesight was weak or impaired. I know this may be painful, and your memory most likely will be hiding any negative memories from you. Our memory tends to try to protect us against past experiences which were painful, frightening, or frustrating. But the only way to work through those memories and the tension which they caused is to remember them and accept them. This is the key to the emotional aspect of vision recovery and health, as well as general spiritual and physical health.

Don't feel you have to write down the "whole story" in this session —just make a beginning. Stay open to memories about this period, and they will come at their own good time, perhaps even in dreams (which you should write down whenever they seem to relate to your vision). Begin this process of recovering these memories now, and expect to continue the process for as long as it takes to fully work through the past experiences and tension caused by them.

SESSION EIGHT

a. Whole-body Exercises

This is an exercise to be done several times during the next few days to compare the physical appearance of your eyes at different times. For the first day, get up before doing the wake-up massages and look at your eyes in the mirror. If you're highly myopic, get close to the mirror so that you can do this without glasses.

First of all, notice how the area around your eyes looks. Can you see tension or strain in your eyebrows, forehead, cheek muscles? Are your eyelids relaxed and blinking, or tense, or tired-looking?

Now look at the whites of your eyes. Are they bloodshot or pure white, off color perhaps? Be aware of the curve of your corneas. Look closely at your iris. What colors do you see? Is your pupil open wide or closed quite a lot?

Now look right into the blackness of your pupils. What do you see?

Finally, ask yourself if you can tell anything about yourself by the "expression" in your eyes? How are you feeling? Do you like looking at yourself, or do you tend to want to look away and stop the exercises? Be honest, accept your feelings, but continue to look regardless, blinking and breathing.

After exercising, look at your eyes again. Can you tell any difference? Would you recognize yourself by looking at a picture of your eyes alone? What qualities make your eyes unique? Is there any feeling of energy emanating from your eyes?

As you go about your day, look at other people's eyes and ask yourself what it is about different sets of eyes that expresses so much about that person's personality and current emotions. Your critical, analytical mind might find itself at a loss for answers, but your intuitive, feeling self will begin to get a hunch, and it is that hunch which will grow into a deeper understanding of how your eyes are a very real expression of your deeper self.

Look at your eyes again later in the day. People have been looking at them all day, but you usually have no feedback as to how your eyes are expressing your feelings, desires, fears, needs. So use mirrors often to begin to get to know yourself visually, from the outside in.

Just before going to bed, pause for a minute or two and look at yourself with no thoughts—just meditate on your eyes while you breathe. Then, in bed with eyes closed, visualize your eyes and see what feelings come to you as you do this.

b. Eye Warm-ups

Hopefully the sun is out when you're ready to do this session. If not, you should probably wait for a sunny day. The warm-up can be done without sun, but the main event does require sunlight.

Indoors or in the shade, close your eyes and imagine that bright sunlight is shining directly on your closed lids. How does it feel? Imagine that you're lying on the beach on your back with your eyes closed. The sun is out and shining down on you. Do your eyes welcome the intense brightness, or do they contract and feel pain and have to be covered with sunglasses or your hand because the light is too intense?

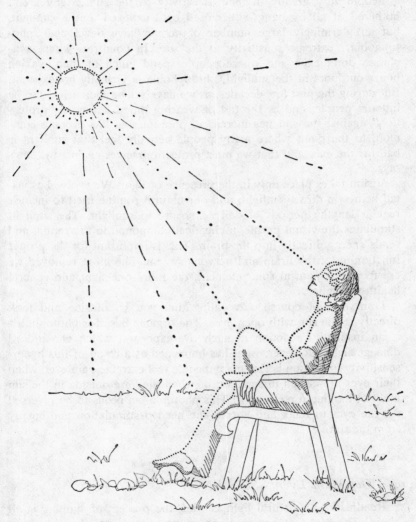

Sunning

People vary greatly in their sensitivity to the sun. Many aren't bothered at all by lying with closed eyes exposed to the sunlight, but an alarmingly large number of people have developed "photophobia," extreme sensitivity to the sun. In countries where sunglasses don't exist and where people spend much of their waking hours outdoors in the sunlight, photophobia is virtually nonexistent. But during the past few decades, as we have grown increasingly to be indoors people, and as the fad of wearing tinted lenses as "protection" against the sun has increased, photophobia has become common, to the point where many people actually feel that sunlight is bad for the eyes and that we must protect ourselves against the sun's rays.

Vision takes place only in the presence of light. We evolved as visual beings in direct sunlight, and our natural routine used to include regular lengthy periods of daily exposure to sunlight. The sunlight stimulates the visual purple, a chemical compound in the retina, and sends energy directly into the brain. This is important for the proper functioning of the brain and nervous system. The more removed we are from our natural solar element, the more our sight and general health will suffer.

I am not, of course, advocating that you go outside and look directly at the sun with open eyes. The organic base for photophobia is an instinctive reaction to such overexposure, which can indeed damage sight. However, what has happened as a result of this hypersensitivity to the sun is that many people feel extreme pain even when their eyes are closed in sunlight, or when they are outside in the sun and not looking directly at it. This photophobia needs to be reversed for the eyes to relax and absorb the needed stimulation and energy from the sun.

c. The Main Event – SUNNING

Readjusting to natural light is what the process of sunning is all about. The fact that our eyes are meant to be exposed regularly to sunlight does not negate the very real problem of oversensitivity.

What does the sun do when it enters the eyes? Consider how the body in general responds to sunlight exposure. When you're lying on the beach, your body relaxes very quickly as the sunlight penetrates the skin to the muscles. Sunlight will also relax your ocular (eye) muscles, and at the same time stimulate the retina and the brain. There is no scientific proof that sunning improves vision, except that so many people have experienced vision improvement through sunning. So try it for yourself!

In this session we'll be combining the short swing movements you've already learned with sun exposure. All sunning will be done with the eyes *closed.* I make this point emphatically because I want it perfectly clear that looking directly at the sun with the eyes *open* can indeed cause retinal damage and should never be done, whereas looking at the sun with the eyes *closed* will not harm the eyes.

So with your eyes closed, sit or stand in direct sunlight. Choose a time of the day when the sun is not at its peak intensity if your eyes are supersensitive to sunlight. Naturally, you won't want to overexpose your skin or your eyes to too much, especially at first. Then do slow, short swings for about two minutes.

Move your head as if you were drawing a circle around the sun with your nose, so that your eyes get exposure from all angles. Draw five to ten circles around the sun in each direction. Breathe deeply so as not to tense as you do this. Don't squint if you can help it; squinting increases photophobia reactions. Sigh, yawn, relax your shoulders if they have tensed up. Feel how the sun relaxes your eyes and your mind. Give in to the incoming sensations of warmth, light, stimulation, relaxation. Marvel at how you can relax and be stimulated at the same time. Let the sun's power totally encompass you as you absorb the primal energy of our solar system.

IN BETWEEN

Every chance you get, sun your eyes. Take every opportunity you find to be outside in the sun, without sunglasses. *Only* when you are in snow or on water or on sand where there is extreme glare should you need to resort to sunglasses. The tinted lenses which darken when you wear them outdoors are particularly harmful, since they never completely readjust to indoor light. This is an additional strain on your eyes.

If you are being bothered by the sun's brightness, instead of reacting and fighting it by squinting and fearing a headache (caused by the reaction, not the sun), close your eyes and sun a little.

YOUR EYELOGUE

Continue writing about your past, bringing up any memories which come to mind, even if they aren't about your eyes per se. Getting your memory healthy is important because much of vision is memory based. When we look at an object which we have seen before, the input from the eyes through some harmonic resonance mechanism stimulates all the stored memories of having seen that object or a similar one in the past. What you experience is both your present visual input and your past visual inputs related to the present one.

Often, when people look at an object, they even see what they remember rather than what they are actually seeing. Or they see what they expect to see rather than what is there. Often people who shave their moustache or beard, or cut their hair, are seen by people who look directly at them without seeing the change. Our brain does indeed do our seeing, and memory plays as important a role as present visual stimulation in what we experience visually.

Many people experience flashes of visual memory while doing the eye exercises, as memories which were buried at the time visual tension set in are released through exercising the muscles where the tension was stored. There appears to be a direct link between emotions, memories, and the muscles where tension was generated when the original emotion was felt and then buried. So if you do experience emotional waves of memory while doing exercises, let those emotions flow, even if they are painful. Getting them out will always make you feel and also see better!

SESSION NINE

a. *Whole-body Exercises*

Chronic neck tension is a problem for nearly all of us. The neck is the most delicate and exposed part of the spinal column, and it is also the narrow channel through which all life support flows between the head and the body. Blood flows upward to the head, and nerve messages flow downward to the rest of the body. Any tension in this area will result in over-all lessening of health and vitality.

There seems to be a direct link between neck tension and visual tension. Neck exercises to relieve this tension are a part of optometric visual training techniques as well as of the more holistic techniques. Optometrists, however, usually suggest doing simple neck rolls. Unfortunately, neck rolls without gentle warm-ups can cause more problems than help if the neck is too tense or has a history of injury.

I've taught yoga for a number of years, and from the yogic tradition I've developed a successful series of warm-ups to ease you into neck rolls. If you've suffered a neck injury in the past, you may find you can do all of these exercises except the final neck rolls, but you'll have to judge for yourself how far to go, or consult your doctor. If you simply have an "all-American" stiff neck like the rest of us, just be sure to keep concentrating on your neck as you do the exercises, so as not to push your stiff muscles too far.

Sit on a firm surface with your spine straight but not stiff. Close your eyes so you can have all your attention focused inward on your neck and your breathing. Gently relax your head forward and down so your chin comes to rest near your chest. Take a deep breath and sigh as you relax the muscles in the back of the neck. The stiffer your neck, the more tendency you will have toward holding your breath as you do exercises, and you need to consciously reverse this old "fear habit."

Now, very slowly and smoothly, ease your head all the way up and

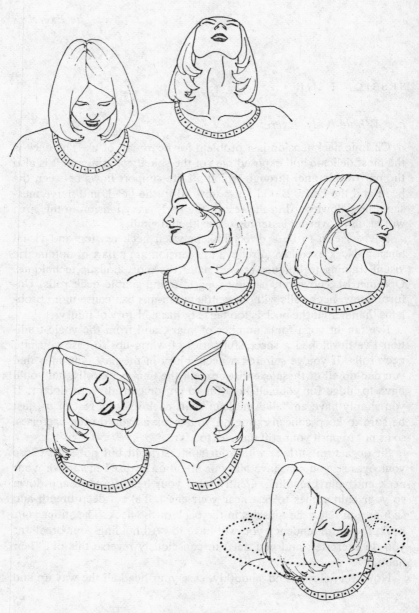

Neck Exercises

back onto your shoulders. Relax your jaw and let it hang loose and open as you breathe through your mouth for a moment in that position. Then go all the way to the chin-on-chest position again, remembering to do all the motions *slowly*. If your muscles seem to have particular spots where they jerk, don't fight to smooth out the jerks—just focus on easing through those spots of tension.

Do this first movement a few times, and then bring your head upright to the starting position. Keep your back straight and slowly turn your head all the way to the right. Feel the muscles in your neck as they stretch and contract. Hold at a maximum stretch which is still comfortable, and then slowly turn your head all the way to your left, with your eyes still closed and your breathing deep. Do this several times, then return to the center and stop.

Now slowly tilt your head to your right, bringing your right ear toward the right shoulder while keeping your back straight. Allow your jaw to drop open, and don't strain too far. Then slowly bring your head back up and tilt it toward the left shoulder. Do this a few times, and then pause in the upright position.

Take a good deep breath and sigh, feeling how your neck is relaxing as you focus on it and encourage it to loosen up. Then slowly extend your head and neck forward and out, like a turtle sticking his head out of his shell. Keep your back straight and feel the stretching at the base of the skull. Jut your jaw out, even though this might feel funny. It will help to relax your lower jaw, which is probably tense.

Now you're ready for a few neck rolls. Let your head hang down in the forward position, and then gently roll your head around to the left in slow motion, remaining aware of your breathing and of any tension spots you encounter. A tension spot feels like a "crick" in your neck. Don't ever push your way through a tense spot. Remember that this is the first time you're doing this exercise, and it will probably take a few times before your neck begins to loosen up in those tight spots.

Roll gently around several times in each direction. Enjoy the movement, rather than push for completion of the roll. If you want to, open your eyes afterward and look at your chart, and see if your vision has improved by doing the rolls.

b. Eye Warm-ups

Now, with your eyes closed and your head perfectly still, just imagine yourself doing three neck rolls completely, fluidly, encountering no tension spots. Then actually do three neck rolls, and see if they don't go more smoothly than the first time you tried them.

Open your eyes when you're finished, blink, breathe, and look into your blur. How's it doing today? Any clearer? After looking a little, do some of the other warm-ups such as edging, short swings, whipping, and the near-far chart, finishing up by palming.

c. The Main Event – *STRING FUSION*

String fusion is the core of your fusion exercise program. It's enjoyable if you don't strain at it, and it works well for both near- and farsighted persons. All you need is a piece of string. The length of the string depends on how good your vision is and how much room you have to work in. For close indoor work you can use a piece just a few feet long, and for longer work, ten feet. Tie large knots along the string every foot, and you're all set.

Tie one end of your string to a doorknob or other stationary object, or better still, have someone hold the other end, and you can do string fusion together. Hold your end of the string up to the tip of your nose. Take a deep breath, blink several butterfly winks, and then focus your gaze on the knot closest to your nose. (If you're farsighted you may need to focus on one farther away to begin with.) What do you see? You should get the illusion of not one string but two strings, and they should appear to cross at that first knot.

If you fail to see two strings, you may be holding the string at the wrong angle. The string should be pointed straight out from you, not off to one side. If you correct this and still don't get the illusion of two strings, you may simply be trying too hard, and through this ten-

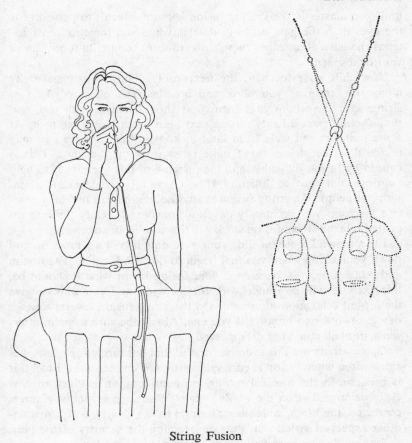

String Fusion

sion short-circuiting the process. Relax, breathe and blink, and allow your eyes to focus on the knot. If you still don't see two strings, you are suppressing one eye. This means you need to go back to the "gate" fusion exercise you learned in Session Three, and work at that until you master it. This string fusion is more difficult to perform for the eyes than the gate, so only do this when you have indeed mastered the gate. Remember there's no rush, no competition, just go at your own speed.

Now shift your focus to the next knot, sliding your gaze easily along the string as you blink and breathe. The effect of the two strings crossing where your focus falls should remain with you, and they should cross directly on the next knot when you come to it. At some point as you slide from knot to knot in this exercise you may notice that the strings don't quite cross right on the knot. This is caused by fusion difficulty, and the purpose of this exercise is to help your eyes correct that difficulty. If you have this problem, and a majority of people do, string fusion is an absolute must in the daily exercise program you eventually develop for yourself. Only through repeated relaxed string-fusion work will this trouble be overcome.

I recommend that you slide your gaze only five or six times up and down your string when you first begin to do string fusion. Then palm and relax your eyes, because if your fusion is not what it should be, this exercise will be rough work for the eyes, and you want to give them total relaxation afterward. Do the string fusion several times a day for two to ten minutes if you can. Always be sure to palm afterward, until all strain has disappeared.

Optometrists use this exercise for children but rarely for adults, because often when fusion is corrected, astigmatism increases. I feel this is because, in the medical setting, no consideration is given to how clear vision will affect the whole person. When one aspect of vision is corrected, the brain, which is still afraid to see clearly, will throw another aspect of vision out, thus maintaining the security of the blur.

So now that you are doing string fusion, you have hopefully grown enough through the previous exercises to accept a recovery of your ability to fuse without having to suffer a regression elsewhere. And even if you do suffer a regression, you are learning step by step that you can grow, that you can make this move into clear vision, and any setbacks will be understood as panic responses of parts of you which need special attention. This is where your eyelogue is so important in the over-all scope of the program, because it will enable you to talk to yourself, to get down on paper how you are reacting to the program, so that you can be aware of those parts of you which need the most attention.

SESSION TEN

a. *Whole-body Exercises*

Another great help in loosening up a chronically stiff neck is the neck and shoulder massage which you can give yourself in about five minutes. Sit comfortably, take a few deep breaths to get centered, and then stretch your arms up toward the ceiling. Enjoy a good stretch with a yawn, then bend your arms at the elbows and place your hands on your back. Put your fingers as far down as they can reach on each side of your spine, with your hands under your shirt or with your shirt off. Breathe deeply and begin pulling the skin away from the spine as your fingers firmly apply pressure outward. This helps open the flow of energy through the spine and relaxes those muscles which run parallel to the spinal cord. Remember to feel from the inside what you're doing from the outside, as if you were meditating on the sensations and encouraging them.

Very slowly work your way up the spine to the neck area, and continue massaging yourself all the way to the base of the skull. Let your head hang forward and sigh as you massage. Do this upward massage several times; enjoy it!

Now, using your thumbs, massage with small circular motions the indentations on either side of the spinal column right below the skull. These indentations will probably be sensitive. Breathe into these spots and allow them to give in to the massage. With your fingers on top of your head, move your thumbs along the base of the skull on either side of the spine outward toward the ears. Notice that you have three sensitive spots on either side, pressure points which need gentle circular rubbing often. Get to know these spots, and massage them

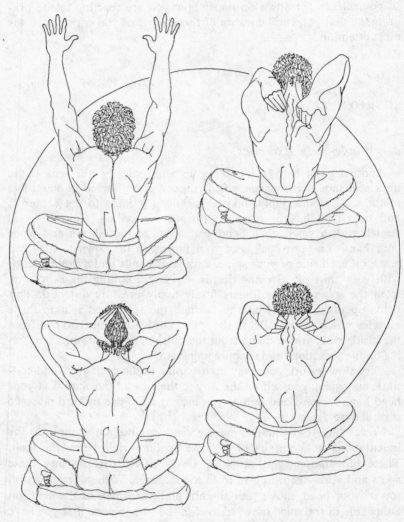

Neck and Shoulder Massage

regularly to promote circulation and relaxation, and prevent head-ache tendencies.

Now continue the massage with your fingers on the scalp, moving the skin on the skull but not running your fingers over the skin. This is also something you should do many times a day for general alertness and relaxation. Then go ahead and give your head a good old scratching massage if that feels good. Yawn, sigh, let your jaw drop loosely, and give yourself a hedonistic relaxation break as often as possible throughout the day. Make faces to relax your face, and end with a full-body stretch and yawn.

b.   Eye Warm-ups

This yogic eye exercise is similar to head rolls, except that you do the rolls with your eyes rather than with your whole head. First of all, go through the neck exercises slowly as indicated in Session Nine, remembering *never* to rush through these warm-ups and neck rolls. Notice how much more freely you can do the neck rolls after giving yourself the neck massage. Combine these two exercises regularly for best results.

Now for the yogic eye exercises. Sit comfortably with your eyes open. Breathe, blink, sigh, and then look up as far as you can, and then down, keeping the head straight. Do this up-and-down exercise ten times, making sure that your breathing remains regular and that you don't tense your face or shoulders.

You can do this exercise quickly or at a slow pace, just fast enough so that your eyes don't fixate on anything going by your visual field. Try doing the exercise both ways, but in the beginning, do it slowly so as not to strain your eyes.

The second movement is from left to right ten times, looking as far as you can see one way and then quickly looking as far as you can the other way.

Now that you've done up and down, and side to side, go diago-

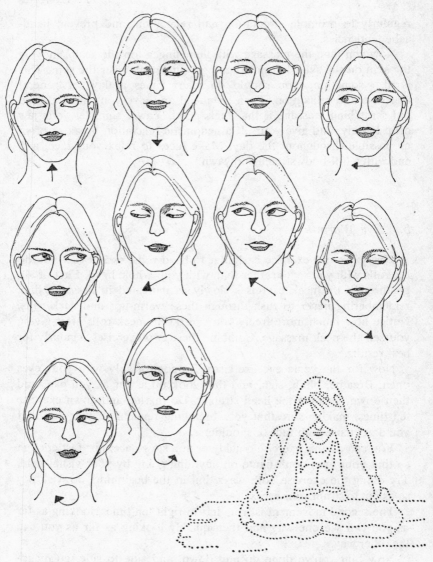

Yoga Eye Exercises

nally, looking up to the left and down to the right. After ten of these, reverse and go up to the right and down to the left. Don't look at anything in particular—just focus inwardly on your eye muscles and get to know them in action.

The fourth step is to make circles with your eyes, rolling them just as you rolled your head in the neck rolls. Start at the top, with your eyes still open, and go all the way around to the right three or four times. Then reverse. Notice that you tend to have spots where you skip, or where your circle gets jerky, just as you did with your neck rolls. Your coordination is not perfect, and there are blocks which will be worked through if you do this exercise faithfully.

Finally, do the eye rolls slowly with your eyes closed. If you find that doing them with your eyes closed is more of a challenge than with the eyes open, you're right in there with the rest of us, and only practice will make perfect.

Once you're through with these yoga eye exercises, be sure to palm. You've strained your eyes, worked them considerably, and they *must* have the relaxation period afterward if you are to benefit from the exercise.

c. The Main Event – SCENE VISUALIZATION

Visualization is an ability of the mind which most people with poor eyesight do very poorly. This is rooted in emotional blocking. If something happened to you as a child, for instance, which you wanted to block out of your memory because it was horrible, frightening, or guilt-ridden, your brain developed the ability to inhibit the recall and visualization of that incident. This in turn inhibited the general visualization ability of the brain. Because much of what occurs in vision is recall of past associations, this inhibition greatly interferes with your seeing. The way to reverse this process is twofold: You need to allow blocked memories to rise to the surface, and you need to exercise your visualization ability by imagining pleasant scenes. We will deal with the release of blocked emotions in a later session. For now, let's enjoy ourselves in a visualization fantasy trip which will both relax your eyes and give them good exercise in the art of visualization. You should probably try to memorize the following scene, have a friend read it to you, or tape it.

All visualization is done while palming, so that the eyes are in complete safety and relaxation. Lie on your back, or sit comfortably at a table with your elbows on a pillow, and imagine that you are lying on a secluded, secure beach. Your eyes are closed at first, as you soak up the sun's warm rays. Feel the sun relaxing your entire body as the sunlight penetrates your skin deeply and enjoyably. You haven't a care in the world, and you sigh out loud as you savor the feeling of warmth, security, and relaxation.

Imagine that you can feel a cool breeze blowing off the ocean, and you can smell that refreshing salt air as you are gently caressed by the breeze. Your skin feels tingly and light, free and contented as you breathe deeply and sigh again.

You can also hear the sound of the ocean, a soft gentle sound broken with an occasional wave breaking in the distance. The sound lulls you into deeper relaxation as your ears follow the intermittent rhythm of the breaking and then receding waves.

After a while, you have a desire to open your eyes (in your imagination, of course, while you continue palming). Slowly you find your lids opening, and you gaze without squinting at the blue sky above you. One small white puffy cloud floats by. You lazily watch the cloud as it floats slowly past your field of vision. For a moment you feel you are the cloud, weightless, moving without effort, headed nowhere in particular.

Then the cloud is gone and you again listen to the roar and hiss of the waves, smell the gentle cool breeze blowing over your body, and feel the relaxing warmth of the sunlight on your skin.

A lone seagull flies overhead, soaring gracefully with wide wings as the wind currents cause it to rise and fall slightly. You notice the bird's white and brown coloring, and its beak which is slightly hooked and yellow. The seagull is high above you, but you can easily see the feathery details of its wings and tail. Watching it soar over you is so effortless and pleasurable that again you sigh and almost feel you are the seagull, flying without effort on the wind.

The seagull soars out of sight. You have a desire to sit up (in your imagination), and you do so, blinking and breathing with continued relaxation and contentment. You look around you with curiosity. You are alone on a small desert island. You remember that your friends on a sailing boat will be back to pick you up in an hour or so. Until then, you are completely free to do anything you want.

The sand around you is purest white. You dig a handful and watch it as it sifts through your fingers. You are aware of its warmth and texture, and marvel at how you can see each individual grain of sand as it falls onto the beach.

Your gaze rises and looks at the ocean surrounding you. It is crystal clear, a beautiful blue color which you can look through right to the shallow bottom of the ocean floor. Brilliant golden brown seaweed sways in a gentle underwater current. A tropical fish with multicolored body swims lazily through the seaweed.

The waves rolling in are gentle. You watch one wave as it builds to a crest, breaks into surging foam, and races for the shore. It hisses along the sand, and a small long-legged bird follows its edge with quick feet and rapid motions of its long slender beak.

As you look around your small island you see a single tree at each end. First you look at the one to your left and notice that it is a tall coconut tree. You look closely with clear vision at the detail of the light brown trunk, and follow the slender trunk up to the dark green fronds swaying high against the brilliant blue sky. There are two coconuts on the tree just below the fronds. One is green, and the other is a ripened brown. You look in the fronds for a monkey, but there is none.

Looking at the other tree, you see that it is a banana tree. Its trunk and long leaves are green, light green, with a single stalk of beautiful ripe yellow bananas.

You look back to the ocean. You feel so content that you make another deep sigh, and let the gentle breeze blow on your face, invigorating you with its salty scent. As you gaze out at the horizon you see a steamship far in the distance. It is a large white ship with two red smokestacks, both issuing a cloud of light gray smoke.

Then, as you look off in another direction, you see the white and red sail of your friend's sailboat heading your way. The sail billows with the wind, and the boat bobs and dips. You can see someone waving to you, a close friend or loved one. You jump up and run along the beach, your body light and full of energy as you race along the edge of a wave to where your friend is beaching the sailboat. By the time you get to the boat your friend is running to greet you with a warm hug.

Allow yourself to stay on the island with your friend as long as you want to, doing whatever you wish, completely carefree and content. In this ideal peaceful situation, your vision is clear and you indulge in soaking up the beauty that surrounds you.

Finally, you say good-by to your fantasy island, promising to return soon. You remove your palms from your eyes, blink gently, and look at your real world with the same sense of openness and relaxation as you experienced on your island.

IN BETWEEN

We're now halfway through. Perhaps you've been involved in this program for three weeks, perhaps three months. I hope that you've felt free to take breaks from your exercises every now and then so that it hasn't become a burdensome task to do daily visual exercises. At the same time, I hope you have been finding time each day to relate with your eyes, to do some exercises, and to palm and relax your eyes afterward.

In these ten sessions we've covered a great deal of ground. I hope you've gone slowly enough to integrate each exercise into your own life, to master the exercise enough to become deeply involved in its meditative aspects. If you feel it would be worth-while, why don't you pause and reread what you've already covered. You will find now that the introductory chapters will take on new meaning, since you have come to understand your own visual personality at a deeper level than when you first opened this book.

Also, if you feel like it, take a few days off from your vision work before going on to Session Eleven. We'll be delving into new realms from here on, as well as continuing with the basic program and introducing new variations to the basic themes. So feel free to take a breather. Enjoy any improvements in vision you have experienced, and get ready for another step.

SESSION ELEVEN

a. Whole-body Exercises

I assume that by now you've developed a whole-body exercise program which is building your endurance, circulation, flexibility, and general physical well-being. For the second half of the whole-body exercises, we're going to be focusing more and more on powerful energy-release exercises, which you can safely do on your own, to energize your being and to discharge emotional pressure which is keeping you tense. Depending on your temperament and needs, you can do these exercises casually and occasionally, or you can make them a major focus in your vision program from here on. By now you hopefully understand the direct relationship between your eyes, your energy level, and your emotions, and can understand why including these more powerful whole-body exercises might be the deciding factor in your visual recovery and general personality expansion.

We'll begin with "Reichian breathing," an exercise which you will hopefully develop as a regular habit to charge yourself with energy, free your breathing from tension, and release any emotions which need to be expressed. It is named after Wilhelm Reich, a psychotherapist who some fifty years ago developed a system of therapy which dealt not just with a person's mind, but also with the emotions and tension stored in the body. Reich's insights into the immutable bond between mind and body, and his techniques for emotional growth through physical exercises, have been a major influence on the development of this vision program. His understanding of the basic energy flow of the human body, and his techniques for freeing up that energy flow when it gets blocked, underlie our vision exercises and give them the power to evoke genuine visual and emotional growth.

Reich discovered that by simply lying on your back and breathing fully and freely you can break through areas of chronic tension so that your life force can flow more naturally and strongly. He used it, of course, in conjunction with other aspects of his therapy, some of which we'll explore in later sessions. For our purpose here it is mainly a way to get the whole body and ocular areas energized so that the vision exercises you do following the Reichian breathing exercise will have a more profound effect.

On a bed or rug lie comfortably on your back with your knees bent, your feet flat on the bed or rug. Close your eyes and begin breathing through the mouth. As you inhale, fill up your stomach and then expand your breath so that the chest fills up as well. Breathe moderately, and try to drop and relax your jaw. Stretch your body a little and get a feel of the surface you are lying on. Then let your complete focus turn to your breathing and to any emotions or sensations which the breathing might be bringing to your awareness.

The most important aspect of this exercise is that you stay in tune with how your feelings and bodily sensations are developing, and allow any expressions which rise to the surface to come out vocally. Reich found that vocal release was one of the finest means of encouraging personality growth, of releasing tension, and increasing the flow of energy. You might wish to close all doors and windows in the room so that you feel free to make any sounds that you want to come out. If you are doing this with a friend, the friend should encourage you to go along with any feelings which arise.

You may or may not have a number of physical sensations develop as you are simply breathing deeply through the mouth. Some people never feel anything except a general sense of exhilaration; others find

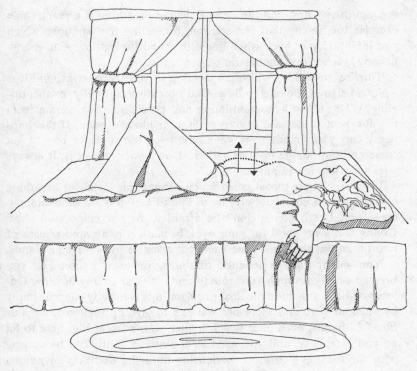

Reichian Breathing

that there are bands of tension in the breathing apparatus which need to be gradually worked through. If your chest and throat are constricted through habitual inhibition of emotions such as sorrow, anger, or fear, this exercise is an ideal vehicle for freeing that constriction and releasing the tension through vocalization of those emotions.

As children, most of us had to inhibit such normal emotions as fear, anger, and sorrow, and this inhibition took physical form in constriction in the chest, the stomach muscles, the throat and tongue, the mouth and lips, and the eyes. Reichian breathing is a remarkable exercise for freeing that constriction, for letting the emotions which you inhibited way back when come out, and for getting your energy flowing in a healthy, unconstricted way again.

Tingling sensations will often develop in your face, arms, and legs —a good sign of the energy flow. Don't breath too rapidly, or this tingling will result in hyperventilation and possible muscle spasm from the unexpected increase in oxygen in your blood system. If this happens, cup your hands over your mouth or use a paper bag to get some carbon dioxide in your system. Don't worry about it; it always goes away in a few minutes.

If you feel your throat constricting against this Reichian breathing exercise, you are probably trying to inhibit a cry or sob that wants to come out. Let it come; don't be afraid to be overcome with sobs. Crying is *always* good for your eyes, because it is a grand release of tension and at the same time excellent exercise for your tear glands.

You might also experience dizziness, or even nausea, as you breathe deeply through your mouth and get your energy flowing. Unless you have a definite medical problem, this is usually caused simply by tensions here and there not wanting to give up their role in your life. Old habits, even ones which hinder your present life, hate to let go and disappear, and you need to coax them gently out by staying with the feelings you are experiencing until the dizziness or nausea lets go and the emotion behind the symptoms comes out. Breathe this way for about five minutes.

b.   Eye Warm-ups

An excellent way to end the Reichian breathing is to open your eyes, blink through the tears if there are any, and look at a friend's eyes or into a mirror for a few moments. Your energy level can actually be expressed through your eyes after charging with Reichian breathing. Allow your eyes to feel "soft" by blinking gently and allowing the emotions to flow through. People with poor vision (and many people with good vision) often have lackluster eyes because the energy flow to the eyes has been shut off. Begin to be aware of this energy flow, and allow your eyes to speak for you. You, of course, can't force this flow. But through Reichian breathing you can increase it, and through eye contact afterward you can express it openly, and this eye contact will be an emotional experience in itself as you continue to let your emotions flow.

c. The Main Event – HAND ENERGIZER AND PALMING

As you have probably discovered for yourself by now, there is something almost magical about the effect experienced simply by placing your palms over your closed eyes. Dr. Bates believed that the differing energy potentials of the hands and the eyes resulted in a flow of current from the hands to the eyes, thus increasing circulation, relaxation, and stimulation in the eyes. The hand-energizer exercise is a means of increasing this charge in the hands, so that the eyes can benefit from palming even more than before.

First of all, rub your palms briskly together. This generates heat and gives your hands a tingling sensation as circulation and energy are increased. Palm for a few moments right after doing this, and see if you like the warmth and energy emanating from your hands to your eyes.

Now take your hands away from your face and spread your fingers wide, pressing your hands together in front of you, thumb to thumb. As your elbows come up, turn your hands so that the fingers point to your chest, and hold that position for a few moments. Close your eyes and focus on your hands as you breathe deeply to increase the charge being generated in your hands. Any shaking which develops in the hands should be encouraged as it is an indication of energy flow into your hands. You might think the mantra "charging" as you do this exercise, to encourage your full concentration. Breathe deeply as you hold this pressure for about two minutes.

Then release and relax your hands, and experience the sensation

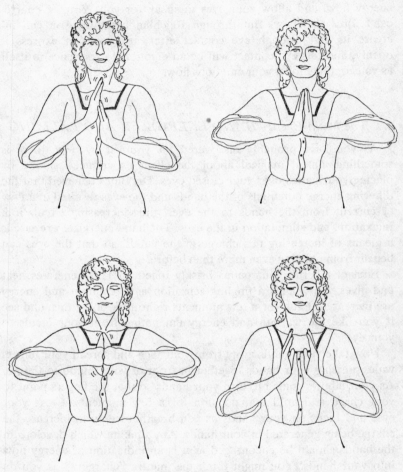

Hand Energizer

you have generated. Hold your hands a few inches from each other, and see if you can't actually feel a flow of energy between them and a "streaming" sensation in the hands themselves, as if energy was passing through them unhindered by the usual tension we all carry in our hands.

Do the exercise again, and then palm. Be aware of the sensation you feel in your eyes, and allow that sensation to flow freely. For your palming meditation, say to yourself, "My life force is flowing, healing my eyes" over and over.

IN BETWEEN

Explore the world of energy and emotional release available to you through the simple Reichian breathing exercise. Experiment with it, see what happens when you do it. Always do it in a room where you won't be disturbed for perhaps half an hour. Let the people in your household know that you are doing an exercise in which you sometimes cry, sometimes shout, sometimes release loud guttural sounds. Tell them that you are trying out an exercise which could have important growth potential for anyone who does it, and encourage them to join you.

If you are lucky enough to have a loved one or friend who will be with you while you do the Reichian breathing, you may feel safer in expressing deep emotions. But don't feel you can't do this alone. Doing the Reichian breathing exercise in a quiet place with a trusted friend, or alone, gives you the chance to temporarily open up to the body's needs and wisdom. If your throat and chest are tense, you need to cry or shout out, you need to release. So go ahead with what your body wants to do, become your body's friend. Gain its trust and develop, step by step with each breathing session you do, a deep trust for it. Because you must trust your body if your eyes are to recover their spontaneous visual health.

YOUR EYELOGUE

Write down how you felt while you took your break following the last session. Hopefully you didn't do any exercises for your eyes at all for a few days. If you didn't take that break, go ahead and take it now! Experience yourself at the new place you have grown to after going through the ten sessions. And write down how you feel about your vision. The eyelogue is similar to the Reichian breathing exercise in that it is your chance to express what you are thinking, what you are intuiting, what you are wanting, etc. Use your eyelogue to let your mind flow freely, as you use the Reichian breathing exercise to let your emotions flow freely. In both cases there is contact with your energy flow.

SESSION TWELVE

a. Whole-body Exercises

The sun-salutation exercise is the best single all-around fitness exercise I know. Your entire body is stretched and toned; circulation is increased; tension is relaxed; energy is increased; awareness is enhanced. You can either do it slowly as a graceful yoga exercise, or rapidly as a vigorous heart-conditioning exercise. Or you can begin slowly and work up to a quick invigorating pace, and then slow down again to "cool off." It's an ideal combination of yoga and aerobic conditioning.

The sun salutation, or "the twelve positions," originated in India as a morning exercise done facing the sun as it rose in the east—thus the term "sun salutation." Doing this exercise outside at sunrise is a very beautiful and invigorating experience, but it can be done anywhere you've room to lie down, and anytime you want to.

Even if you are "fit," you might find some of the twelve positions of the sun salutation difficult at first, because they are coordination and limbering exercises as well as fitness exercises. Approach this exercise as you approach your eye exercises: Accept your present physical state and do only what you can without straining yourself.

Make sure you've enough space to lie down on, then stand straight and well balanced, to realize how you feel physically, particularly your energy flow. Close your eyes for a moment to feel your body and its sense of balance. Take a deep breath and perhaps sigh, and then begin with position one.

One: Exhale (all breathing is done through the nose except when you are doing the postures vigorously) and press your palms together over your solar plexus, pressing down so that the chest or bust muscles are toned and strengthened.

Two: Inhale as you stretch your hands toward the sky or ceiling. Arch your back, tuck your seat under, and have a good stretch.

Three: Exhale as you stretch down and out to the floor, keeping your back rounded. Place your palms flat on the floor on either side of your feet, bending your legs if necessary.

Four: Inhaling, take a long step back with your *right* leg, so that you end up with your right toe and knee on the floor and your head *up.* You should feel a good healthy stretch all along your right side from your chin to your toes.

Five: Holding your breath, step back with the *left* leg as well, so that you end up in what would be the middle of an American push-up. Keep your body as straight as possible.

Six: Exhale as you lower your *knees, chest,* and *forehead* to the floor. Let your seat come up in the air. Any reasonable facsimile of this posture will do at first; it's a rather unique stretching position.

Seven: Inhale as you lower yourself to the floor, and then slowly push up with your arms so that the top half of your body rises up and back. Leave your hips on the floor, your elbows bent a little, and

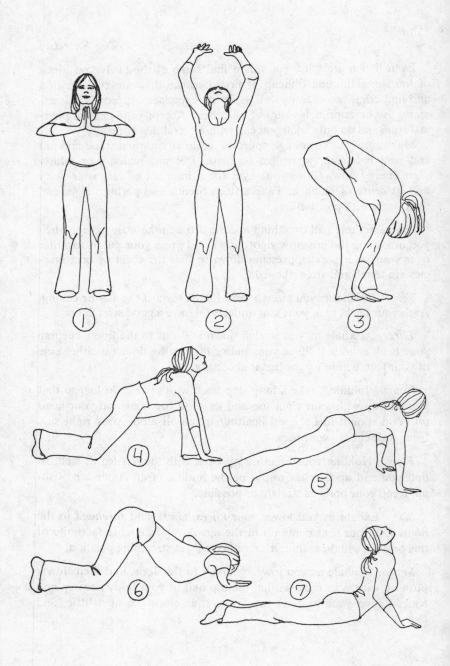

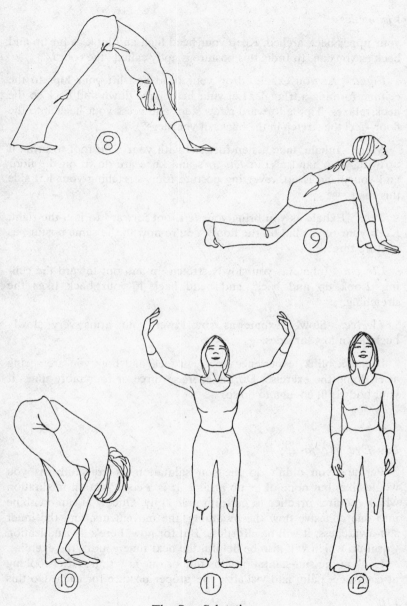

The Sun Salutation

your upper back arched. Keep your head high and look as far up and back as you can. In India this posture is aptly called "the cobra."

Eight: As you exhale, drop your head and lift your hips to the ceiling, forming a triangle. Let your head hang down and back so the neck relaxes. Tiptoe forward a few steps and press your heels into the floor—feel the stretch in the backs of your legs.

Nine: Inhale, take a step forward with your *right* foot to bring it up with your hands. Your *left* toes and knee are down on the floor and your head is up, reversing posture four, stretching your left side this time.

Ten: Exhale as you bring your *left* foot forward to join the right. Keep your palms flat on the floor. You're now in the same posture as posture three.

Eleven: Inhale as you slowly stretch up and out toward the ceiling. Look up and back, and bend back if your back likes the stretching.

Twelve: Slowly exhale as you lower your arms very slowly back down to your sides.

Breathe, blink, experience how you feel, and how you are seeing after doing the exercise. Do the exercise three or four more times if your body is fit enough to do so.

b. Eye Warm-ups

Perhaps you didn't do the sun salutation as gracefully as you would like, but none of us do at first. It is a coordination meditation which requires practice to perform gracefully. Once you can combine into one cohesive flow the breathing, the movements, and the inner self-awareness, it will be effortless. But for now, here's a visualization warm-up which will also be helpful the next time you try the exercise.

Look at the sun-salutation illustrations one at a time. After looking at each one, palm and visualize the proper posture for each. Do this with all twelve postures, and then close your eyes and do the postures yourself, visualizing yourself performing with perfect grace and fluidity. This visualization is a great eye exercise, and imagining yourself graceful will help you to become more graceful in reality.

c. The Main Event – *FLASHING*

While we're working on the sun salutation, here is another sun-oriented exercise. First of all, however, relax your eyes with a few short swings in the sun.

Once you've sunned for a few minutes, stand or sit comfortably facing the sun and we'll do what's called "flashing," a method of sunning which stimulates the chemical layer of the retina known as the

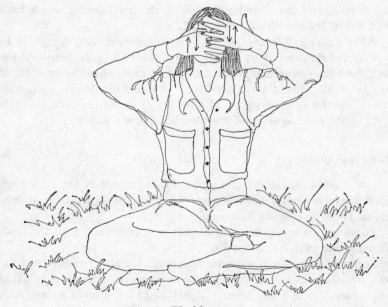

Flashing

"visual purple," the chemical vital to the transference of the sun's vibratory rays of light into the electrochemical energy. Through stimulating this visual purple, you will increase the "muscle tone" of the retina and thus see the world afterward as exceptionally bright and clear, as if it had just been freshly washed.

With your eyes *closed,* hold your hands about three inches in front of your face with fingers spread apart a little. From the elbows, start moving your hands quickly back and forth a little in front of your eyes. The light passing through the areas between your fingers will give a strobelike flashing effect to your eyes and retina, creating a delightful, multicolored effect. Keep your hands shaking and enjoy the visual fun!

Flashing is healthy for any kind of visual problem, or for general preventive eye care. But it is especially powerful in helping aging eyes recover their youthful vigor because of the stimulation of the visual purple, and the stimulation also of the iris muscles which tend with age to freeze with a narrow pupil.

After flashing, it is always best to do some more long swings, or to just sit and do some short swings, lazy eights or whatever, around the sun. And then palm and allow the eyes to experience the contrast of blackness after the stimulation. Like everything else in life, such contrasts give the eyes strength and a feeling of expansiveness and vitality. Finally, palm again until complete blackness returns.

IN BETWEEN

Pause and again make sure you are doing regularly the earlier exercises which should have become a part of your daily vision program. These include the following.

Palming is a must, as often as you can, combined with whatever visualization exercises you enjoy.

Swinging is another must, because both the short swings and the long swings help loosen up eye tension so much, along with relaxing other parts of the body. Short swinging and *visualization* go naturally together, as do palming and visualization.

Accommodation, particularly with the whipping exercise and the regular use of a near-far chart.

Sunning regularly is vital. Get out in the sunlight as much as you can, go on hikes, bike rides, play frisbee, and other sports which get you outside, and, of course, do the actual exercises for sunning.

Fusion exercises are crucial for training the eyes to work as a team. Not only do people with blurry vision have trouble with fusion, but so do many people with "normal" eyesight. This can result in headaches and eye strain in either case. It seems that the first thing the brain does when it doesn't want to see something is that it throws the fusion of the stereoscopic eyes out of whack, with one eye refusing to look at an object even when the other eye is doing as ordered. The two hemispheres of the brain are quite different, as research is showing, and it appears that one side of the brain can control one eye, and the other side the other eye, creating infinite potential for fusion trouble. You must work regularly to get your eyes working together, and keep them working as a pair throughout your life. The string-fusion exercise is the finest exercise. Looking through the gate (Session Three) is also good, and we'll be focusing on fusion quite a bit in upcoming sessions.

Centralization is a skill necessary to develop sharp, detailed vision. Do remember to edge *all the time,* to help with centralization and to get the eyes shifting, also to develop the habit of taking in as much information about an object as possible, so as to give the brain enough input to put together a clear, complete picture.

Whole-body and energizing exercises, especially the Reichian breathing exercise, which could prove invaluable to your visual and over-all well-being.

YOUR EYELOGUE

Write a critique of your vision schedule. How often do you do exercises? For how long? How regular are you in doing the exercises? Do you do a well-rounded exercise program or do you tend to forget or avoid one or more of the seven areas? Do you enjoy the exercises or are they really "work"? Do you feel resistance from some part of you that tries to keep you from doing regular exercises? Are you aware of any new positive habits you are developing visually? How's your breathing coming?

Now think about how your habits have changed with regard to wearing your glasses or contacts. How do you feel about them right now? Put them on if they're handy: How does the world look through them? If your eyes are improving, your glasses are now too strong for your eyes.

You can either say you've reached a point where you don't need your glasses, except for movies and night driving. Or you can admit you still need them often, and therefore must either get out an old pair of weaker prescription lenses, or go to the optometrist for a weaker prescription.

However, don't expect too much support for your eye improvement program. Sadly, many eye doctors still believe the old myth that eye exercises won't hurt you, eye exercises won't help you, eye exercises will just waste your time. Even if you do encounter such an attitude, you are still the client paying for a service, and it is within your right to receive the kind of prescription you desire.

If you go to the optometrist, here are some thoughts for you to consider before, during, and after the visit.

It is obvious that my emphasis is on personal responsibility for vision care, rather than for placing that responsibility on the costly shoulders of the medical profession. But a periodic visit to an optometrist or an ophthalmologist is necessary to give you progressively weaker prescriptions as you need them, and especially to check for any signs of glaucoma, cataract, and other eye diseases which the medical profession can treat.

First of all, do you go to an optometrist or an ophthalmologist? The difference is this: An optometrist, like a dentist, has four years of training in his specialty, but no M.D. degree. The ophthalmologist is an M.D. who specializes in the eyes. You might think that, therefore, a genuine M.D. would be your best choice, but this is not necessarily the case. An ophthalmologist deals primarily in eye diseases and spends much of his time doing eye surgery and dealing with specialized drugs and radical vision problems. An optometrist is more oriented toward the regular vision problems of refractive error, fusion difficulty, and so on. When he detects a "medical" disease which requires drugs or surgery, he must send you to an ophthalmologist, but otherwise he is the man (or infrequently the woman) who deals on a day-to-day basis with regular vision problems, and will often have much more experience in fitting corrective lenses and dealing with vision exercise programs. Also, the optometrist will usually be less expensive, more available, and probably more open to your particular approach to your eyes.

What exactly do you want in this prescription? You want glasses which give you about 20/40 vision, just adequate for passing the driving test. The aim is to get your eye muscles doing as much of the vision work as possible, with as little dependence on the corrective lenses as possible. The eye doctor will try to tell you you're hurting your eyes by doing this, unless he's keeping abreast of the new approaches to vision. But you can insist on what you want, and if he won't give you the reduced prescriptions, go elsewhere. And *make sure* that you feel you're getting adequate reduction based on your normal present vision, rather than on a nervous reading at the eye doctor's.

If you're nearsighted, bifocals can be of help to you. They allow your lens to relax properly for close work. Whatever, it's important to stay relaxed during the exam so that tension doesn't result in a temporary poor reading. This means going on a "good" day, preceded by some relaxation exercises and remembering to breathe and blink while you are there.

Write down your own feelings about visits to eye doctors and other experiences you've had related to wearing glasses. How do optometrists and ophthalmologists treat you? Do they fully explain their tests and results to you? Do you indeed get nervous visiting their offices? Do you want to be free of your glasses and rid of the corrective lenses hassle once and for all? Feel that desire and let it propel you as you do your exercises!

SESSION THIRTEEN

a. *Whole-body Exercises*

Alexander Lowen, the founder of bioenergetics and one of the foremost leaders to emerge from the Reichian school of thought, has developed a number of exercises which are powerful in energizing your body and getting you in touch with your basic life force. The exercises help you to "let down" if you are feeling "hung up," they help you "get your feet on the ground" if you're feeling "out of touch."

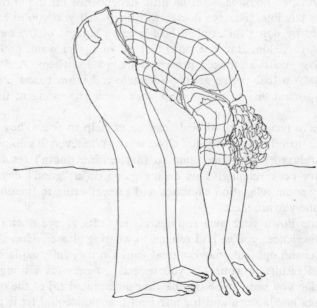

Grounding Flop

Such metaphors give only a suggestion of the real power of these simple exercises. The one you'll learn here is known as "grounding."

First of all, stand in loose clothing or without clothes and slowly bend over so that your fingers touch the ground or floor. Let your head flop. Don't put any weight on your fingers; they're just used here for balance. Turn your toes in, with the weight of your body on the balls of your feet, and experience the stress as vibration passes through your body. Breathe deeply into your diaphragm rather than up in your chest. After about a minute, your legs will have a tendency to vibrate "out of control," and this is exactly what you want to happen!

If you don't feel a good vibrating stretch in the backs of your legs, straighten your knees somewhat and raise your heels off the ground to increase the stress. Hold this posture for about a minute, breathing deeply through your mouth. Feel your contact with the ground, feel the energy beginning to shake and vibrate through your legs and body, and go with that vibration. The sensation can be absolutely remarkable. You might even feel the tips of your fingers vibrating as they lightly touch the ground. If the vibration becomes intense and emotions arise, feel free to make sounds in this position, to get in touch and stay in touch with your body as it releases energy and tension and generates a charge of vibratory flow. Hold this position for about two minutes.

b. Eye Warm-ups

This new exercise, like "seeing one thing best" and the edging exercises, is designed to help you with centralization and mobility. It is called "counting," and is a form of scanning. You can begin right now by looking up from this book, and with your eyes scan for corners of objects in the room. Count to yourself if you like, or just notice corners as you see them, and then move quickly in search of another corner of an object. (As with edging, be sure to keep your head and eyes moving together.)

Try doing this with a particular color or a particular curve. The more you do this, the more your eyes get into the game of scanning and regain their ability to zero in on specifics. Remember to blink and breathe. If you're walking on a city street, count mouths, eyes, hats, black shoes, brunettes, beards—anything you want. Just let your eyes enjoy the sensation of seeking details, finding them, and moving instantly on to more details. This is an exercise you can do virtually anywhere, because nature repeats itself so often and gives you plenty of room to play your game.

c. The Main Event—VISUALIZATION and MEMORIZATION

As I've mentioned earlier, people with poor eyesight are sometimes poor visualizers and also poor memorizers of visual detail. This exercise will help you to develop a better visual memory. What you will do is to look carefully at something, and then close your eyes and remember what you saw.

Choose an object in your environment or open a magazine or book to find a picture which strongly attracts you. Take in the details of the scene and edge the objects or forms within it, scanning and blinking, breathing and relaxing as you absorb.

Then close your eyes and remember what you saw. It is important to be aware that visualization is not something that happens in the eyes. Many people who are poor visualizers think that visualization is actually an ocular experience, and look at their eyelids for the picture show. In actuality, visualization takes place deep in the brain, not in the eyes.

As you recall the details, list them verbally, in a clear, strong voice. At first you may only remember the major details of a scene or picture or object. Now open your eyes and look at the room or the picture again, and scan for details. Did you remember it correctly? Or are you surprised by the difference in what your memory and your eyes recall? As you scan this time, pick up color, shapes, details, but don't "try" too hard, just enjoy looking closely at the object or picture. And then close your eyes again and see what you remember. Repeat this process as often as you want—the more times the better.

IN BETWEEN

Look about you as if you had to memorize your surroundings. Just looking with this memory recall in mind will make you so much more aware of what you are seeing.

Inability to remember goes hand in hand with poor vision, so you must fight against this tendency to shut out any memory flashes from your present awareness. This visualization exercise is a great loosener of memory in general. Do it often!

SESSION FOURTEEN

a. Whole-body Exercises

In Session Thirteen you bent over forward in the basic Lowen grounding posture. We're now going to reverse that posture with what is called the "Lowen bow." This exercise will be of great help to people with tension across the pelvic and lower back areas, a condition which inhibits the flow of energy throughout the body. It also further establishes the feeling of being solidly grounded. As with the Reichian breathing technique, it can be done anytime, but will greatly enhance a vision session if done just before beginning the exercise.

When fully performed, this exercise brings flashes of visual clarity to some people. You will be breathing deeply through the mouth as you maintain the stress position. The energy generated by breathing into this stress often breaks energy blocks which free the eyes of chronic tension and inhibition of emotional expression.

Begin standing with your feet about eighteen inches apart, and toes slightly turned in. Bend your knees slightly, tuck your hips, and arch your back. Make fists, and place them knuckles up against the small of your back, on either side of your spine right above the pelvic bone. You'll probably find that you're pressing into tense muscles. This posture will help those muscles relax.

Breathe deeply through the mouth and into your diaphragm as you experience the stress this posture generates. Focus on an object in front of you, feel your body begin to vibrate from the stress, and allow your legs to give in to this vibration as it grows. If you are

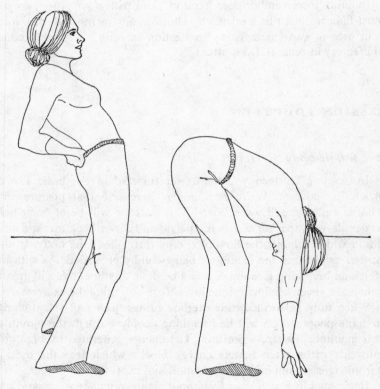

The Lowen Bow

habitually tense, you will feel more stress in this posture. Go into that stress, experience it deeply, make guttural sounds of pain as much as you want to, to help relieve your system of the pent-up tension. Continue to breathe deeply and experience yourself as you give in to the stress and allow your body to vibrate and your voice to express your anguish at the chronic tension in your body. Let it all out and be done with it!

Stay with the posture until you can't hold it any longer, twenty breaths or more. Then hang over in the grounding exercise you learned in the last session. *Always* finish the Lowen bow with its reverse posture. Hanging limply with your knees bent a little and your fingers touching the floor, focus on your breathing and on the vibratory sensations in your body. Then slowly stand up and breathe deeply as you reflect on the experience you just had.

If your lower back, thighs, or other parts of your body feel strain afterward this is an indication of where you're packing the most tension, where you need to do the most work. You should find that these two exercises will release tension in the lower back rather than increase it, as your knuckles knead into those muscles under stress and bring energy to them.

If your lower back really aches, now or anytime, lie down on your back, bring your knees up so that your feet are flat on the floor, and press your lower back against the floor, alternating between pressing and relaxing. Breathe deeply, allow the pelvis to move freely, sigh, let your back sink into the floor, and rest a few moments. You might also bring your knees up to your chest and roll gently first to one side and then the other, to give the lower back further release from tension. Have your arms out straight at the sides, palms down, for this, and turn your head in the opposite direction from where your knees and legs are going. Breathe deeply in the stomach and sigh as your lower spine releases and relaxes.

b. *Eye Warm-ups*

A combination of palming and sunning called the "sun sandwich," will greatly stimulate vision. This is a combination of palming and sunning. You simply sun for a minute or so, doing short swings or long swings as you wish. And then you palm for an equal amount of time. Anywhere from five to ten alterations is good, always ending with palming. This is a way to both relax and invigorate the eyes at the same time. Myopes and presbyopes alike, both of whom have somewhat frozen iris muscles, will benefit greatly from this alteration between darkness and light because the sun sandwich keeps the pupils changing size. Do this often if your eyes tend to have difficulty in adjusting to abrupt changes in lighting.

Feel tense right now? Make a face and shake off the tension as you learned to in this session. Do this often when you feel your face is wearing a mask. Keep yourself out in the open!

c. *The Main Event—THUMB FUSION*

Thumb fusion is similar to finger-shift fusion except that instead of holding one finger farther away from the other, you hold your two thumbs the same distance from your nose, starting with the knuckles almost touching.

Your arms should be as far out as they go in front of you, with your thumbs up from fists and close together at first. By slightly crossing your eyes and focusing in space about halfway in front of the thumbs, you can create the illusion of a third thumb between your two thumbs, as shown in the illustration.

If you have trouble getting this third image, have a friend hold a pencil or finger at that halfway point between your eyes and your thumbs, where your eyes should be focusing. As you look at the pencil or finger, have it removed, and the phantom thumb should appear. Remember to breathe and blink, and hold the image for a minute or

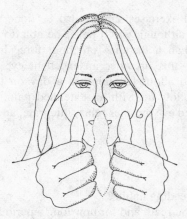

Thumb Fusion

so while you edge that middle thumb and see how clearly you can fuse the two images which are generating that third thumb. If your eyes feel at all strained, remember to palm for a few moments before going on.

Now you're going to generate a phantom thumb by looking in the distance beyond your thumbs. Give it a try. There! For a real super-fusion exercise, change your focus from in front of the thumbs to beyond them into the distance. Go back and forth like this as quickly as you can. Feel that great workout your eye muscles are getting. At first it will be a real effort to pull off, but the more you do this, the more effortless it will become.

A final variation on the thumb fusion which is healthy and also fun involves moving the thumbs. Focusing in front of your thumbs, slowly move them apart while you continue to hold the phantom thumb in place. As the phantom starts to go fuzzy or blurry or to break into more thumbs, give up and start over. Yes, the phantom thumb will shrink as you move your real thumbs farther apart. At first you'll only be able to go a few inches apart, but soon you'll get to six or nine inches if you practice regularly for a few days or a week —some people can go up to several feet.

Visionetics

Both these final exercises should also be done with the focus beyond the thumbs, although you'll never be able to hold the phantom image for more than a distance of about three inches between the thumbs. However, this provides an excellent eye stretch, especially for myopes. Spend about ten minutes a day on thumb fusion, and then be sure to follow up with an extended palming vacation to let those well-exercised eye muscles relax, integrate, and learn.

IN BETWEEN

What are your reading habits?

How often do you read, and for how long a period?

Are you a "book junkie" who reads to escape, as many of us nearsighted people do?

Do you read for long periods without looking up?

Do you palm regularly while taking reading breaks?

Do you read in good or bad light?

What kind of material do you read, and are you reading under stress, as in studying for exams?

Do your eyes ache after or during reading?

Do you breathe and blink regularly, or do you stare and breathe shallowly?

In your eyelogue, write down the answers to these questions. Take your time, think about your reading history, and make any notes of interest.

When you sit down to read, pause for a moment to consider your emotional state. If you are tense, your eyes are going to be contaminated with this tension and naturally you're going to experience eye strain when reading. So if you're tense, breathe deeply and palm a few minutes before reading to get relaxed. Or do some whole-body release exercises.

Then consider why you're reading the book in hand. If it is for pleasure, fine. If it is for schoolwork or other reasons that place demands on you, be aware that tension is a factor. Pause now and then to do some whole-body exercises and palming; get up and move to start your circulation going, and remind yourself that your eyes are your sense organs, not just work horses.

For all reading, if you blink and breathe regularly, your eyestrain will be reduced greatly. Even if you're reading a thriller that keeps you tense emotionally, remember that your eyes are suffering from this tension even though you might be enjoying the excitement.

Look up from the printed page occasionally and look into the distance, to let your accommodation muscles take a breather as you shift your focus from near to far. Use this pause to do the near-far exercise in one form or another. Edge outlines in the distance as you take your "breather." Be aware of how your eyesight changes as you continue reading.

Lighting is very important; the more light (without glare), the better, in most cases. I often use a 250-watt reflector spot bulb for night reading. And, of course, reading with the sun or daylight over your left shoulder is best.

Try reading without your glasses, unless you are so near- or farsighted that you simply can't see the words. If you want to exercise your eyes while you read, hold the book in your blur zone now and then.

A final suggestion is to do the neck and shoulder massage you learned in Session Ten while you're reading. Often your neck will become stiff while you read, and you need to correct this. Also, it will feel good!

In general, try to focus more on satisfaction with what you are doing rather than on getting finished with the work. When reading, take your time, look up and enjoy yourself in the midst of your reading, rather than read at breakneck speed. If something is worth reading at all, isn't it worth pausing and savoring regularly?

SESSION FIFTEEN

a. Whole-body Exercises

"The woodchopper" is one of the most powerful warm-up whole-body exercises. If this one is within your physical ability—and it should be unless you suffer from severe back trouble, high blood pressure, or related problems—you'll find it extremely powerful and energizing for the whole body, and also especially invigorating for the eyes. So much energy will be brought to your ocular region that, after the exercise, you should feel a strong tingling sensation in your eyes.

Before you begin, do the stretching exercises you've learned, some upper body and hip rotations (Session Seven), and the two grounding exercises. Now, with loose or no clothing, assume a comfortable, wide-legged stance that affords you a good sense of balance. Breathe deeply and pause to check on the clarity of your vision before doing the exercise.

Then, holding your arms straight in front of you, pretend that you're holding an ax with both hands. Feel the weight of the ax head and adjust your shoulders to that weight. Tuck your hips in as if preparing for a swing of the ax to cut some wood in front of you.

Lift the ax toward the ceiling over your head, and inhale deeply through your mouth as you do so. Throw your head back, start to exhale, and swing the ax down in front of you with a great exhalation, allowing your arms to swing all the way between your legs. Make any sound with which you want to punctuate this swing, a karate-chop shout or any powerful expression to go along with your vigorous swing.

Then allow your body to swing back up into position to take another swing, inhaling as you go up, exhaling strongly on your down swing. Begin this exercise slowly and easily, and then allow your

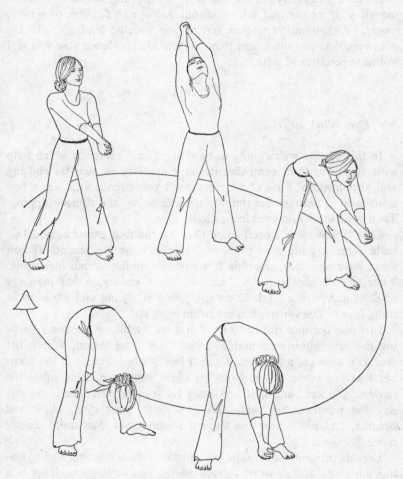

The Woodchopper

body to accelerate the pace and increase the intensity of the down swing until you really get into the flow of chopping wood, of expressing all your power and self-assertion. Allow any feelings of power, anger, or exhilaration to flow out of you vocally! End up swinging with complete abandon, and then pause and experience how you feel in this supercharged state.

b. Eye Warm-ups

In this session we're going to be doing "fun" exercises which help with all skills, from centralization and mobility to near-far shifting and visualization. First of all, why don't you edge a little, do a few short swings, perhaps the thumb-fusion exercise, and some whipping. Then palm until your eyes feel rested.

Good! Now, you'll need some dice for the first exercise, and two balls (tennis, golf, even oranges or apples) for the second. If you don't have any dice save this first exercise until you can buy some. Your dice should be of the black on white variety, rather than the colored translucent kind. Begin using one at a time and work up to using four or five when it is not a strain to do so.

Just toss the dice out in front of you on a table or the floor, keeping the toss within reasonable distance for your vision. Watch the dice as it bounces and spins. When it finally stops, glance at the number that has come up, and quickly close your eyes. Remember the number you saw, and if it was fuzzy let yourself visualize it clearly. Say the number out loud, and then open your eyes, blink and breathe, and see if you don't see the number of dots more clearly now.

Do this for quite some time with just one dice, relaxing and enjoying the visualization work as well as the open-eye game. This is a great exercise for loosening up stiffening presbyopic (farsighted) lenses, and if you're nearsighted, focusing on the visualization and memorization will help to bring about maximum vision improvement.

Add more dice to your routine when you're ready to take on an extra without straining or getting tense at the new variable.

When you feel you've done enough, palm for a while to relax the eyes.

c. *The Main Event – BALL TOSSING and JUGGLING*

The old axiom of "watch the ball" has great significance in vision training. Regardless of whether you're playing frisbee, tennis, baseball, basketball, golf, or whatever (Ping-Pong is great for the eyes!), if you focus on the ball as it comes and goes, you're doing wonderful mobility and accommodation exercising. You want to watch the ball *all the time.* People with poor vision very often don't do this, and it shows up in their eyesight as well as in their game scores.

Sit or stand comfortably with one ball (a tennis ball is probably best but use what you have at hand) and just toss the ball into the air, head and eyes moving. Watch its ascent and descent with total concentration. Toss it with one hand, catch it with the other, and transfer the ball back to the original hand for the new toss. Breathe and blink, and juggle for about five minutes.

This is a simple and yet such effective exercise for weak eyes. I do it as a meditation, watching the ball as I breathe deeply, allowing my complete awareness to focus on the ball as it participates in the game of getting tossed up by me, and pulled down by gravity, around and around in the up-and-down game.

If you want, you can use two balls for added fun, going as fast as you can while remaining calm and graceful in the game. Do this whenever you have little breaks, tossing anything up and watching it. And afterward, of course, *palm!* If you don't palm you'll be wasting half of your effort by not relaxing the eyes afterward.

IN BETWEEN

Get out and play frisbee as often as you can. The frisbee is perhaps the finest throwing object for visual exercising because it is sensitive

129

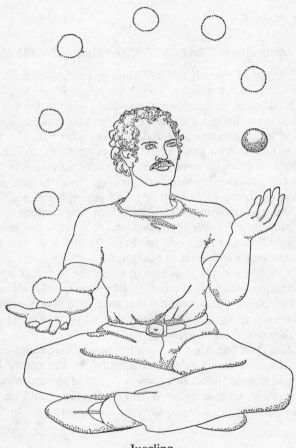

Juggling

to the wind and moves unexpectedly up and down, this way and that, forcing your eyes to stay alert all the time. It also moves with a graceful speed which varies, depending on the throw, providing an infinite variety of curves to watch with your eyes. Of course, baseball, catch, and other ball-oriented sports and pastimes are fine too.

The most important thing is that you get out regularly and get your body moving in coordination with your eyesight. Your heart and circulation will be helped as you help your eyes. I encourage adults to make friends with a youngster in the neighborhood and play frisbee with him/her, as well as playing with other adults. Watching a youngster learn how to throw a frisbee will give you insight into what your eyes need to do to become spontaneous.

Watching a tennis match is also excellent eye exercise, if you keep your eye on the ball all the time. Be sensitive to all the moving activity in your day, and as often as you can, follow it with your eyes, whether it be birds overhead or healthy bodies going by!

YOUR EYELOGUE

It would be a good idea, after making notes on your present visual program and experiences, to consider your general habits during a regular day. What do you do? Are you active or sedentary? Do you walk whenever you get the chance, or take the car or bus or subway short distances to avoid exercise? Do you feel good and loose in your body when you walk, or are you tense and stiff? Is your diet healthy, or are you a junk-food junkie? Make any other entries about your daily habits, just to gain a perspective on yourself. List anything you can think of—how often you make love, if at all, how long you sleep, what drugs you take, and so on.

I might offer a few thoughts on nutrition at this point. If you don't eat well, you can expect nutrition to play a negative role in your vision. Theories blaming nutrition on poor eyesight have not been proven, but there are certain foodstuffs and vitamins which do have definite positive or negative effects on vision. For instance, there seems to be some correlation between insufficient protein and myopia. Although the research thus far is inconclusive, if you have a low-protein diet you may want to increase your protein intake.

If you are photophobic or oversensitive to sunlight, it may help you to increase your vitamin B intake, although raw sunflower seeds are excellent for doing this "organically."

Circulation necessary for good vision can be augmented through taking vitamins C, E, and lecithin. If you don't get enough sun, vitamin D is also important. I am not a great fan of vitamin-popping fads, but since our natural foods seem to be lacking in many vitamins, taking pills seems a necessary "evil" at times. So, depending on your diet, keep your vitamin level adequate; most importantly, try to keep your diet full of fresh vegetables, fruit, and nuts so that you get a maximum amount of natural vitamins from your food.

Vitamin A is usually the vitamin associated with eyesight. There seems to be a connection between vitamin A deficiency and night blindness, so it would behoove us to keep our vitamin A intake up, naturally if possible, with pills when necessary. Keep in mind, however, that too much vitamin A is toxic, so don't take over 5,000 mg a day.

SESSION SIXTEEN

a. Whole-body Exercises

You've probably noticed that a number of the whole-body exercises are designed to get your head down low and reverse the pull of gravity on the ocular area and the head. The shoulder stand, a gentle yoga position, is perfect for this. You will not only get blood into the head where you need it for vision health, but you will also stimulate your thyroid gland. The thyroid gland controls your metabolism, and it is so often actually squeezed and constricted by tension in the throat that doctors are beginning to realize that tension causes thyroid and low-energy problems. Eyes and metabolisms which are aging will particularly benefit from daily upside-down shoulder-stand exercising, but regardless of your age, getting upside down is one of the easy shortcuts to good health. The shoulder stand is easier to do than a headstand, and it reduces the strain on the neck which a headstand often generates. Begin by lying comfortably on a firm surface—a carpet with open room around you is best. With loose or no clothing, bring both legs up perpendicular to the floor. This in itself is a good exercise.

Then, press against the floor with your elbows and lift the bottom half of your body into the air, catching yourself at the hips with your hands. There you have it, the half shoulder stand! You should be comfortably supported with your hands on your hips. If your feet are directly over your head, that's okay, but it's best to have them back over your hips.

Here in the half shoulder stand you'll be able to feel if you're ready to go on up to the full shoulder stand. If the blood rushing into your head is too intense a feeling this first time, or if being this far upside down is making you feel dizzy, just breathe deeply in this posture and remain in it until you feel ready to come back down. Be aware of the feeling in your eyes as you breathe. You can hold this posture for up to five minutes, but if you feel dizzy, come down immediately.

If you're going on up into the full shoulder stand, walk your hands up your back toward your shoulders, bringing your body up as straight and as tall as you can. The straighter you get, the more you're massaging your thyroid. Usually you'll feel this as a slight constriction in your breathing. Bear with it unless it's too much, breathing as fully and as easily as possible while holding the posture. Three to five minutes of this is ideal, but don't push yourself the first few times.

Focus for a moment on your feet way up there where your head usually is. How do they feel? Reflect upon the fact that the head and eyes are usually above the heart and thus gravity pulls the blood down away from them when you're upright. This yoga position, which along with the headstand is considered the ultimate rejuvenator of physical postures, should be included in a daily program of holistic fitness and body awareness.

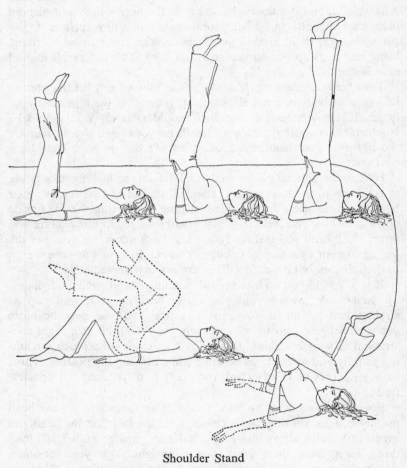

Shoulder Stand

To come down without crashing, bend your knees to your chest, shift your arms so they are supporting your weight on the floor, and gently ease your back all the way down. Rest awhile when you're down, and see how you feel and see: pausing each time after doing such an exercise and focusing on how the exercise has affected you is half the learning process.

If your lower back hurts afterward, bend your legs to your chest and rest that way. A Lowen bow and the rag-doll hanging position for grounding would go well either before or after this.

Playing soft music is a help for doing this posture, to allow your mind to relax completely and flow with the posture.

b. Eye Warm-ups

To combine edging and counting exercise with an enjoyable card game, you might want to play solitaire. This game, like tossing dice, promotes mobility and mind-eye interplay at a rapid level, with the excitement of the game keeping the eyes moving rapidly.

Play the game as you ordinarily would, but see if you can alter the way you look at the cards. Shift your eyes back and forth over the cards, first by moving your whole head as you scan, and then by just moving your eyes. Go back and forth between these two ways of looking. Breathe and blink, and if tension develops in your shoulders give yourself regular massages there and ease up a bit on the game. Remember to enjoy the present experience rather than being half in the future.

Also, count hearts or spades, etc.; edge the cards and face-card figures, and in general do all the good healthy things for your eyes that you've been learning to do, catching yourself when you stare, hold your breath, don't edge, etc. And enjoy!

c. The Main Event – HEALING VISUALIZATION

Recently, there has been remarkable evidence from cancer research that meditative visualization can bring about retardation in cancer patients, and genuine reversal in a considerable number of them. When healing visualization as a regular habit is applied to visual recovery, the success is much more noted than with cancer. Once you learn this technique, you can also apply it for colds and other illnesses in which the strength of your body's resistance to disease is the crucial factor in recovery.

What you are going to do first is to visualize your eyes, and then to visualize your eyes undergoing the changes necessary for better vision. As you alter your brain's image of your eyes, you will obviously be giving your brain a direct opportunity to send messages to the eyes to alter the eyes also. This exercise works from the brain out to the eyes, from the source of the problem to its visual effect.

Palming is the vehicle for doing this exercise. As you palm, breathe deeply and focus on your eyes. Feel them in there. Visualize the eyes with their muscles (an aesthetic visualization rather than a surgical one works best) and feel your present contraction.

If you are nearsighted, visualize your present eye shape with the muscles that go around its middle squeezing it out of shape, so that it is elongated from front to back. Visualize your cornea under stress and buckling under the tension to produce astigmatism. And visualize the ciliary muscles which control the lens as being spasmed. Imagine the blood vessels which feed the eye area squeezed so that the blood isn't flowing freely through the vessels.

If you are farsighted, visualize your eyes as being squeezed from back to front by the muscles behind the eyeball, squashing the eyeball forward and throwing the focus beyond the retina rather than on it. Visualize your lenses as stiff, unyielding, needing more blood and ciliary muscle activity to get it back in shape.

Now encourage your visualized eye to relax, talking to it, coaxing it, and watching as the muscles slowly begin to get the message, to loosen their grip and ease off a little. Bit by bit, you can see the bands of tense muscles loosening and relaxing, responding to your request and your assurance that everything is okay. Tell them that you want them to continue to do their job of moving the eyes as you look in different directions, and you want them to continue to hold the eyeball in shape, but that the shape needs to be more responsive to the interplay of the eyes and the brain.

Sigh every now and then as you allow your entire body to relax along with the eye muscles and lenses. Feel the blood vessels opening wide and allowing the life-bringing blood to flow freely through the eye areas.

Now, with your eye shape looking healthy and unsqueezed, feel the focus of light beginning to move toward the retina. Watch those ciliary muscles relax and loosen up, altering the shape of the lenses so that the focus lands perfectly on the fovea of the retina.

Imagine life-giving energy coming into your body with each inhalation, flowing up through your eyes and expanding your eyes to their natural shape. As the energy flows through, it heals the tense muscles and frozen lenses, and then with your exhalation carries any tension and toxins out of the body. It is such a soothing, organic, natural way to breathe, bringing energy in as you inhale, and letting tension leave the body as you exhale. The energy can either be felt as a soothing breathlike flow, or perhaps as a stream of vibrating, healing light which cleanses your visual organs and leaves them alive, vibrating with energy, and able to remain relaxed and healthy once the exercise is over.

Now breathe deeply, take your hands away from your eyes, blink softly, and look around you. Some people experience flashes of perfect clarity after doing this healing visualization. If you do experience this flash of clarity, breathe into it, and allow the clarity to spread throughout your body as if it was energy itself, bringing light and relaxation to your entire being.

Don't try to hold on to such a flash, let it come and go, welcome it when it comes, say, "See you later" when it goes. If you didn't experience such a flash, don't judge yourself or the exercise for not working the first time. In fact, some people never have flashes, but do improve their eyesight steadily, nevertheless. The flashes of clarity after the exercise are bonuses, the real growth visually is what happens as you're visualizing, because you are step by step, every time you do this exercise, developing a new image of your eyes for the brain to work with, and sooner or later the contact is going to be made between the brain's new image and the muscles in the eyes, and the flash will occur.

I recommend that you get up and go for a walk afterward, allowing your eyes to be free to do what they want without placing any demands on them. If flashes of clarity come as you're walking, breathe energy into that clarity but don't hold on; just enjoy!

IN BETWEEN

Now that you've learned the healing visualization, you will want to do it at least five times before deciding if it works for you or not. Take plenty of time with this session, and do the exercise at different times of the day to see when is your best time for visualizing. Research seems to indicate that we have ninety-minute cycles, during which we move regularly into a more reflective state, and then a more active state. See if you can be sensitive to when you "feel like" doing this visualization meditation, and do it for perhaps fifteen or twenty minutes.

But also carry this ideal visualized image of your eyes with you all the time, seeing it whenever you think of your eyes and encouraging your brain to get the picture translated into muscle talk that reaches the eye muscles and actualizes your visualization.

SESSION SEVENTEEN

a. *Whole-body Exercises*

A major personality trait of most myopes, and many farsighted people as well, is a tendency to suppress anger inside. Often, people will hold anger so deeply buried that they aren't even aware that they have any. This tendency is developed early in life; the eyes of such people are usually lackluster, and these persons are afraid to let anyone really look into their eyes deeply for fear that the unacceptable anger would be seen.

Such blocking of a powerful emotion will take its toll on the body. There is a theory that hyperopes become farsighted in order to somehow escape from seeing their own body, which contains the anger they are afraid to express or have no acceptable way of expressing. This pair of exercises is very important in releasing pent-up anger and frustration, in getting energy flowing out of the eyes again, and in relaxing the ocular muscles which have been tensed because of buried anger.

Pounding can be used by anyone regardless of whether or not he has a vision problem, but Dr. Charles Kelley has developed a method of pounding that is especially valuable for myopes, as well as anyone with vision problems. Regardless of your visual condition, give this exercise several chances to work for you. It is a completely safe and acceptable way of venting powerful emotions, and as such is extremely valuable to us all. If you react to this exercise by feeling you aren't an angry person and don't need exercise to vent anger or frustration, you are probably exactly the person who will benefit most, so be game and give it a go!

There are two ways (at least) of doing this exercise. One is with a towel, and the other is with a tennis racket. First I'll describe the towel-pounding technique. Take a bath towel and fold it so that you end up with a long, round, inch-or-two thick flexible pounding instrument. It is best done by rolling the towel across its width.

Sit on your heels, on a rug or with a pillow under your knees. Breathe deeply through the mouth for a few moments with your eyes closed, feeling energy rising into your shoulders and arms. Keep your gaze fixed on an imaginary target, while slowly raising the towel up over your head with both hands holding one end of the towel. Take a deep breath, as you exhale come down, and hit the floor in front of you with the towel, "breaking" your wrists as you do so to avoid hurting your hands. Take another deep breath, raise your towel and your body up again, as shown in the illustration, and as you exhale come down again with a good solid thump on the floor in front of you.

Continue doing this, slowly at first and fairly gently, but increasing

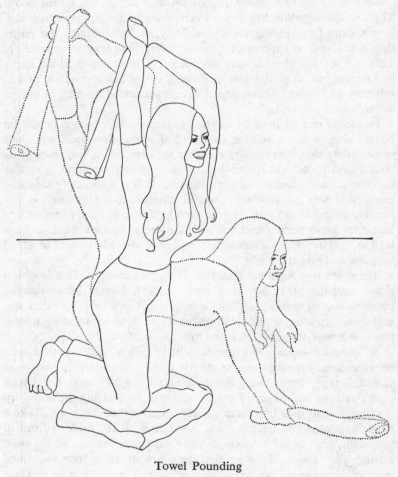

Towel Pounding

the rapidity and strength of the towel pounding with increasing rhythmic intensity until you let yourself go and get completely into the feeling of hitting as hard as you can, with all your energy and emotions behind your hit. Allow any sounds to come out of your mouth—a loud karate-chop shout or a "Take that!" or a mean hostile sneer, any sound which wants to come out should be allowed to do so. Then, when you feel finished, breathe deeply to catch your breath. Keep your eyes open, focused on a specific spot in the distance (eye contact in a mirror is best), blink gently and allow your eyes to feel "soft" as the energy flows through them.

This simple hitting exercise will quite possibly run head-on into cultural taboos you were brought up with. Perhaps you were severely disciplined for expressing anger as a small child. Perhaps you were taught that you were to be kind and sweet always, never aggressive and hostile. Women were taught that anger was an unacceptable emotion, and men often keep their anger deeply buried because they're afraid that they cannot control their physical hostility.

This exercise is a compromise between inhibiting a genuine emotion and doing someone else (or yourself) actual physical damage. If you allow yourself to regularly release pent-up emotions of anger, hostility, rage, or frustration through towel pounding, you will be doing yourself a vital service without in any way hurting anybody. So please do give this exercise a chance. For your eyes' sake alone it is important. If you feel anger and hold it in check and try to hide it, your eyes will be tense and blocked emotionally in the attempt to cover up your genuine emotions. If you are frightened and generally shy and afraid of violence, this will help you find your inherent strength and sense of self-assertion so that you won't have to be afraid any more. You will know that you are strong and can respond with anger when it is called for.

A variation on towel pounding, which I like very much and which often works much better than towel pounding, for me and for people I work with, is pounding on a bed with an old tennis racket.

The tennis racket will make a great powerful sound, and you will feel your energy with great intensity. Keep your eyes on a spot you are hitting, keep your vision in focus, and if you want to, imagine some-

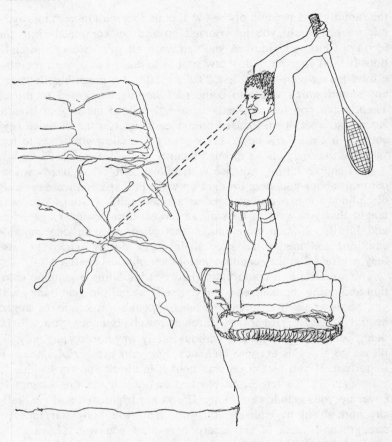

one there whom you feel angry at, either in the present or someone in your past. Raise the racket up over your head and as you bring it down, say, "Take *that!*" Or even say words you might usually keep yourself from saying, such as "I hate you!" or "Leave me *alone!*" A simple *"no!"* is often most effective, said with each hit and building to a rapid climax.

b. Eye Warm-ups

In conjunction with towel pounding, it can be helpful to have a friend sit about five feet away from you as you pound and express your anger. After pounding, force yourself to seek eye contact with your friend and maintain it as you catch your breath. This might at first be very difficult for you to do, but it is important that you allow someone else to see you as angry or upset, and for that person to accept that part of you. Even more important, if energy flows freely while your eyes are thus directed, your eyes have the best chance of adjusting properly for that distance (in this case, to your friend).

You can also set up a large mirror to watch yourself as you pound, seeing how you look and how your eyes change as the energy starts to flow out of them. Even without another person present or a mirror, keep your eyes focused on an object in the room. During this eye contact, blink gently and allow your eyes to become "soft" after having been "hard" in anger. Realize that if you never express anger and feel hard, your eyes will also never be able to relax and feel soft and open, because you are having to be guarded to hide the hard emotions. Have soft eye contact with your friend if he/she is there, and in general feel the flow of positive postaggressive energy flow through you!

I should mention in concluding this discussion on towel pounding and tennis-racket pounding that you will not necessarily feel aggression and anger when you do the exercises described here. You might feel, for instance, just the opposite emotions—weakness, hopelessness, anxiety, or fear. As you pound, your defenses might win out and try to immobilize you so that you won't get in touch with your anger. If this happens, if your breathing becomes tight and depressed and you feel temporarily weak or dizzy, just sit there and breathe into those feelings, accept them for the present, and reflect on what this defense against expressing anger might mean to you personally and to your eyesight in particular. Don't be upset with yourself for not being able to do the exercise "correctly." As with all these exercises, the aim is to get in touch with yourself, and to grow from there.

c. The Main Event – *PATCHING*

Pause for a moment, examine your blur, and see how it is doing this morning. How would you compare it to when you looked into your blur during the first session of this program? Close your eyes, palm, and meditate for a moment on the growth you've experienced during these seventeen sessions. How do your eyes feel now? Are they more relaxed as you palm? Are you more in touch with any tension which is continuing to remain? Can you visualize your eyes as healthy and free of unnecessary tension, as you began doing in Session Sixteen?

Now, keeping one hand in place, take away the other hand and look at the world through just one eye. What kind of vision do you have in this eye? Relax, breathe and blink, and get to know that eye with its unique perception that is not necessarily like the perception in the other eye.

Palm a moment with both hands, and then remove the other hand so that you can look through that other eye alone and see what its vision is like. Just look, don't compare right now with the other eye.

Now cover one eye and then the other, comparing the vision in each to the other. Which eye is "weaker"? Which eye do you feel needs the most work? Once you have made that decision, palm and focus on that eye, and let it know you want to help it recover its natural healthy state.

One way to help it become stronger is to wear a patch often over the other eye. You can buy eye patches at most drugstores, and they are valuable aids in vision exercising. Put the patch over your good eye so that your "bad" eye has to do all the work. Then edge, blink, scan, whip a little, and end up palming awhile.

Do the near-far chart (Session Six) or play solitaire with this one eye and then palm again. Take special care to palm after a patching exercise, because that weak eye has really had a workout.

Now and then put the patch over the weak eye and let the stronger eye have a good workout too. But, mostly, keep it over the strong eye. You can wear this patch around the house regularly for a while to give that weaker eye the feeling that it has the responsibility for your total vision during those periods. This will encourage general recovery of that eye, which usually lets the other eye do most of the work.

Swings, long and short, are valuable when patching. The one eye

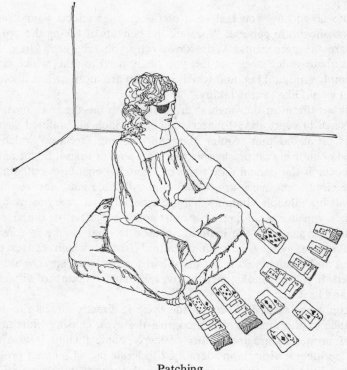

Patching

that is looking will really have to confront its bad habits and will adapt to take a more equal part in stereoscopic vision.

With both eyes, after patching and palming, do string visualization and thumb fusion, to see how the eyes are now working together.

YOUR EYELOGUE

Make a list of all the prescription drugs you've taken in the last year, noting how many, how often. Now make a list of all the non-prescription drugs you take with any regularity (at least once a month).

Write down how you feel each of these drugs affects your vision and your health in general. What are the benefits of taking the drugs, what are the detriments? Write down why you take each drug. Be honest about which ones you feel you really need to take, which ones you simply enjoy taking, and which ones you are more or less hooked on, but would like to stop taking.

Perhaps the most detrimental drugs to vision are the ones most of us use nearly every day: tobacco, coffee, alcohol, and refined sugar.

It is estimated that regular cigarette smoking (tobacco which is inhaled) can bring on presbyopia ten years sooner than it might naturally occur if the person didn't smoke. Smoking cigarettes cuts down on the circulation necessary to maintain a flexible lens, and nicotine also eats up valuable vitamins that are especially necessary as we age. Whether you are a smoker or a nonsmoker subjected to the smoke pollution of smokers, the irritation caused by that smoke is considerable to the eyes. Any such unnatural irritant which causes eye redness and scratchiness is certainly bad for the eyes, and should be avoided. If you do smoke, be sure you take extra amounts of vitamins C, E, and lecithin.

Alcohol has several effects on the eyes. It directly affects the performance of the muscles which control the eyes, causing blurriness, loss of proper focus, and failure of stereoscopic fusion. It also reduces peripheral vision considerably. Moderate use of alcohol probably does little harm to eyesight, and the temporary relaxation might even help the eyes. But the over-all, long-term effects of the drug on the body are detrimental to good health, and use of alcohol should be kept to reasonable levels if you are concerned about helping your eyesight. When alcohol becomes an addiction, it obviously reflects a general problem of the whole being, and the eyesight cannot help but be negatively affected by such an addiction. Because alcohol eats up B and C vitamins, you should supplement your diet if you drink much.

Sugar, refined (white) sugar in particular, is a drug which during the past fifty years has been accepted into our diet with gigantic "success" and also with disastrous effects on our over-all health. A hundred years ago, sugar was a simple condiment, used like other condiments in small quantities. But these days, sugar is in almost everything that is preprocessed and serves as America's most popular artificial stimulant. It goes into the blood stream and temporarily increases one's energy, but it places rugged demands on the body, makes it run at an unnatural speed, and then, having depleted the body of its natural energy, runs the body into its reserves by continued stimulation. The long-term effects of this artificial stimulation lead to a general deterioration of the body.

The "low" that follows a sugar "high" reduces vision performance considerably, causing blurriness and vision failure, especially at the mental level. You might very possibly double your flashes of clear vision and your general vision improvement if you cut out as much sugar as you can from your diet for a month. I highly recommend trying this.

Coffee is another drug which artificially stimulates the body. When coffee and sugar are used to supplant and replace good food intake, the body naturally suffers on all fronts. So when you feel the "need" for a candy bar, a Coke, or coffee, why not stand up, stretch, do a Lowen bow and then the rag-doll hang, breathe deeply, and see if you can't take care of your energy needs without resorting to drugs.

Marijuana can have a positive, if temporary, effect on vision. It affects the muscles which dysfunction in glaucoma, relieving the problem when ingested. Since marijuana is the only present "cure" for relieving glaucoma, there is a movement underway to make it an acceptable prescription drug for this purpose. This effort has been helped by the recent case of the United States vs. Robert C. Randall, in which Mr. Randall's physician was given permission to obtain marijuana from the National Institute of Drug Abuse for the purpose of alleviating the symptoms of his glaucoma. Also, the state of New Mexico has just passed a law that makes it possible for hospitals, upon court order, to treat patients with marijuana if they so request.

The focus of this book is on holistic awareness of how your body responds to its environment. Regarding drugs, I would only say that if you remain sensitive to how a drug affects you, you will know whether it is healthy or detrimental to your vision, and based on those perceptions, you can make your own decisions.

SESSION EIGHTEEN

a. Whole-body Exercises

I would like to offer several variations to add to the Reichian breathing exercise, so that this can become a more total exercise when done alone.

On your back, after having breathed deeply for several moments with your knees bent and your eyes closed, begin lifting and dropping your legs as if you were actually running. This is a basic bioenergetic charging exercise which will increase your Reichian breathing experience considerably as it brings your breathing to a deeper and more rapid pace and gets your whole body in action.

As you're "running" with eyes closed, say, "I want to get away," several times. Then change this to "I want to run away," and say that as often as it feels good. Your running might very well take on a light free energetic flow when you feel you're running away. Say out loud, "I'm running away!" and allow yourself to just take off in your imagination, making good your escape.

You might want to use other phrases, such as "I've *got* to get away" or "Leave me alone." "You can't stop me" works well also.

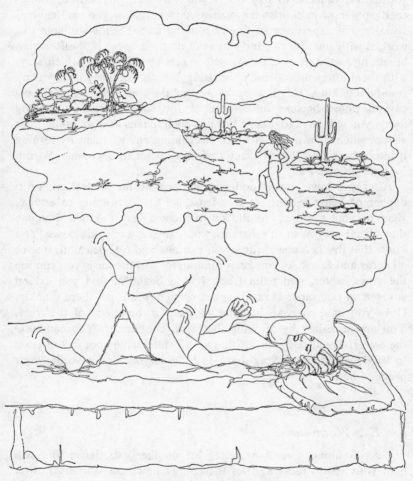

Reichian Breathing (Variation)

The point is for you to give in to past desires to flee when in reality you didn't; you had to stay where you were unhappy, afraid, threatened, somehow held prisoner against your will. Now you can feel and visualize the experience of finally running away! Some students I've worked with run and run and run (still on their backs in the Reichian breathing position, of course), with a new-found energy which stays with them afterward, a feeling of being able to run away if they can't stand something. This is a basic need of the spirit, to feel it can escape if things become intolerable. If you can't escape by running away, you will have to escape through such means as developing poor vision which does away with the threatening environment by turning it into a blur, and that is exactly what we want to overcome. So run for your vision's life!

After you have run a good distance and no longer feel you're in danger of being caught by past fears, let go of running to escape. Keep up your running, but allow it to become easy and light. Imagine that ahead of you in the distance you can see an idyllic oasis. You know that this is a place where you can rest and feel peaceful, free of all cares and fears. As you keep running toward the oasis you can see the grass, water, and palm trees. It's so beautiful that you extend yourself in one more burst of speed so that you'll get there quickly. Once you have arrived, imagine yourself in the shade of the trees. You are refreshed by drinking the clear, cool water. You can taste the water. Then, see yourself finding a comfortable spot in the grass to lie down and rest. Stay there as long as you like, savoring your peace of mind.

b. Eye Warm-ups

Let's combine several exercises for another experience that will help your vision relax and let the energy flow. On your back after doing some Reichian breathing, focus on your eyes (closed), your neck, and your pelvis. Your knees are bent and your feet flat on the bed or rug (a firm surface is best).

Exhale, contract your body, flatten your back against the rug, pull your chin down, and imagine you are looking down at the center of your being, with your whole body tensed as you push air and tension out.

Then relax, inhale deeply, look up toward the top of your head with eyes closed, allow your back to arch, your stomach to inflate, your pelvis to tilt freely, and your body to expand as you take in a charge of energy and air.

Do this several times, as long as it feels good, but at least three to

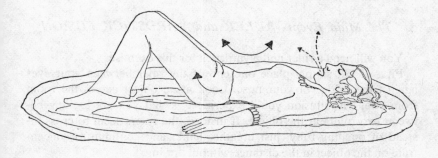

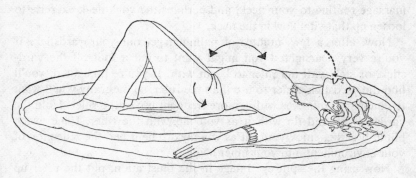

The Pelvic Rock

five minutes. You should experience a positive flow of energy, sexual or otherwise, through your body while you become relaxed and energized at the same time. It's important to realize that these two qualities go hand in hand, being relaxed and energized. The opposite to both of them is being tense and contracted.

As you do this "pelvic rock" exercise, allow your eyes to feel the contraction and then the relaxation, the dispelling of tension and the inward flowing of relaxation and energy.

c. The Main Event – RULER and YARDSTICK FUSION

You will need a ruler and a yardstick for this exercise.

First of all, simply place one end of the ruler between your eyes against the bridge of your nose. Look at an object across the room from you. The illusion you'll experience is that you are looking between two rulers at the object. If instead, the rulers seem to cross instead of opening fully, just breathe, blink, and continue to concentrate on the object in the distance without "trying."

Edge around the room, looking between the two rulers as you do so, and give your eyes a good session of edging, moving your whole head naturally. If you feel tension in your neck, remember to do the massage routine to your neck, and perhaps the yoga neck exercise to loosen up that vital flow in the neck.

Now, after a few minutes of palming, get out your yardstick. If you're very nearsighted you might want to cut a foot off the yardstick, or stay with the ruler to begin with. If you're farsighted, you'll find the yardstick easier to use than the ruler, so naturally you'll want to challenge your eyes with a more frequent use of the ruler. Hold the yardstick up and do with it as you did with the ruler. Edge away, blink, breathe, enjoy yourself as you absorb light and the reflection of your environment into your inner being.

Now using the split-eye image in the illustration, put the ruler up in place between your eyes as before, and then put the book up

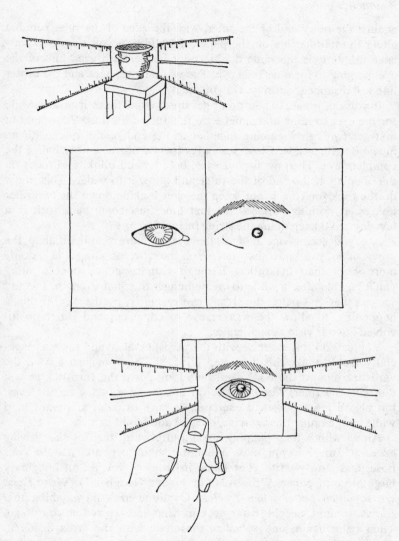

Ruler and Yardstick Fusion

against the other end of the ruler, with the edge of the ruler running along the middle line on the paper. The illusion you should experience this time is the same double-ruler image, with each half of the eye merging to form a single eye. The two outer images and the center line will disappear entirely. Do you see it?

If you do, great. If not, don't get upset; sometimes it takes awhile for the eyes to relax and experience this fusion illusion. You might at first get two rulers coming together at the end of the ruler with an image on either side. Close your eyes for a moment and visualize the complete eye. Then open your eyes, breathe and blink, and focus on the opening at the end of the ruler and allow it to widen. This might do the trick for you. If not, keep the eyes looking down the two ruler images. If nothing happens the first time, just come back to it in a few days, and keep doing the string fusion!

Are you seeing one half of the eye as more dominant than the other? If so, you know that the eye on the corresponding side is doing more work than the other. Through visualizing and concentrating you'll be able after a while to create images of equal strength. I would suggest that you patch the strong eye regularly, by the way, if this is happening, to allow the weaker eye to come out and get more involved in your vision experiences.

You can do this exercise with the yardstick also, and myopes especially should make this final step. Place the book against a wall, the yardstick against the book, and then look down the yardstick as you did with the ruler. The effort to do this is more taxing on the eyes, but also a more powerful exercise. Be sure to palm afterward, and while you're doing this exercise, breathe and blink!

Along with a long palming session afterward, try this short-swing exercise. Imagine you have a paintbrush or pen attached to your nose, and slowly write your name in front of you on an imaginary large piece of paper. Write *relax* in cursive (longhand). Write *I can see so much better when I relax*. Continue to write anything that comes to mind, keeping your neck moving and relaxed as you do so. Then palm again, and visualize the circle with the cross inside it. Think of the cross as a plus sign reflecting your increased fusion and visual relaxation.

IN BETWEEN

As a reminder of the importance of swinging to help the eyes recover their natural vibratory scanning ability, stand up and do the long swing with your eyes open, watching the world go by as you slowly swing your arms and shift your weight.

Now close one eye and very gently, while you swing, bring one hand up and lightly touch the closed eye as you continue with your swinging. You will feel that eyeball moving rapidly under the eyelid as it continues to participate in the activity the open eye is involved in while swinging. This activity is what swinging is designed to encourage, until the eye recovers its spontaneous habit of always looking with this vibratory movement. This is not an exercise to be practiced, but rather a demonstration of how swinging affects the shifting of the eyes.

YOUR EYELOGUE

The kind of lighting under which you live and work can strongly influence the way you see. Direct sunlight is best; fluorescent is the most detrimental. Now write down, as you consider your environment, where you encounter fluorescent lighting fixtures as opposed to regular lighting fixtures. At your place of work? In your home or workshop? At the doctor's office? Banks? Your school or your children's school? What percentage of your average day is spent under the influence of fluorescent lighting?

This is an extremely important consideration. Fluorescent lighting is virtually taking the place of the regular light bulb in our country. It uses less energy and eliminates a lot of glare, but the negative effects far outweigh the positive:

1. Fluorescent lights throw off virtually no shadows and give a low, diffused level of illumination. Because the eye sees mainly through the interpretation of contrasts, of shadows against whiteness, with lighting that eliminates shadows, the eyes must strain to see. A fright-

ening number of people in their thirties are developing myopia, and this one factor of working under fluorescent lighting is often the only one that has caused the development of poor vision.

2. The fluorescent buzz is another problem, particularly with the lighting in older buildings. The nervousness of factory workers, which leads to tension, headaches, and then fatigue, is partly caused by this constant irritant directly over their heads.

3. The flickering of the fluorescent tubes is another menace. These lights vibrate at a particular pulse which interferes with the different vibratory patterns of our brain. This jarring irritation to our nervous system can result in more tension and fatigue to tax the eye muscles and eye/brain communication.

4. Probably the most far-reaching detrimental effect of fluorescent lights is that they don't give off the full spectrum of light we normally receive from the sun. It has been demonstrated that animals need the sun's full-spectrum light to stimulate the endocrine and pituitary glands for proper performance in regulating our bodies. In 1973 the Environmental Health and Light Research Institute in Sarasota, Florida, conducted such a study on first-graders. One group of children was observed under cool-light fluorescent tubes (the type commonly used in schools and offices), and another control group studied under shielded, full-spectrum lighting. Those children in the classrooms using the standard cool-light tubes exhibited nervous fatigue, irritability, lapses of memory and hyperactive behavior. Both groups of children were then kept under full-spectrum lighting, and the behavior of the first group began to improve within a week.

SESSION NINETEEN

a. Whole-body Exercises

In dealing with chronic tension in the body, we've seen how inhibition of basic emotional expressions can create tension throughout the body, with a resulting decrease in clear vision. An emotion you should now explore is the final expression we will be dealing with at the whole-body level.

This is the emotion of revulsion, of wanting to spit something out, of wanting to express your distaste for something. When this gut-response reaction to something in your environment is inhibited, the entire face and throat and also the stomach must somehow mask the true feelings. The eyes, through which so much of our expression emanates, are intimately caught up in this inhibition, and therefore suffer directly from such chronic repression of distaste or disgust.

The exercise for releasing this mask the face has created is simple: it's one you did as a child until you were forced to stop. Right then is when you started developing your frozen mask, and you have probably developed it into quite an unconscious art—not letting people know when you don't like something, when you want to reject rather than accept something which is being forced on you one way or the other.

First do this alone if you wish, and then with a friend. At first you're going to feel a little embarrassed, because you're probably conditioned *never* to make faces like the ones I'm going to suggest. But go ahead—you'll be surprised at how very much of a relief it will be to let this side of your personality out. Especially if you think you don't have this side to you at all, do this exercise a number of times.

Stand in a room where you're free to make any movements and noises you want. Imagine a horrible taste you can't stand, and express your repulsion at just the thought of having that taste in your mouth. Make a "yech" sound, raising your upper lip in distaste, so that your nose gets squeezed up as if the very thought of the smell offends you to the core. Stick your head out from your shoulders and act like you're spitting something out of your mouth with distaste, giving all the sound effects you can muster to express yourself.

Now go a step further and stick out your tongue and allow yourself to go "blaaaa" with vehemence as you shake your head and almost shiver down your body at the thought of something that is so "yuckey" it repulses you with disgust and disdain. Bellow out your repulsion so the world knows how you feel.

A few people might vomit when they do this, and should back off from the exercise. But go ahead and gag, fire off all those muscles which have been holding that throw-up feeling in check all these years. You'll be amazed at what a relief it is to gag on some vague past memory which you had to swallow at the time.

Afterward, be aware of how your eyes got lubricated, stimulated, and charged with energy. When I work with a group doing vision training, and finally get them over their inhibitions and into making faces at each other and hamming it up, the room becomes electric with energy being released, and I see eyes brighten up after the individuals are allowed to let that disgusted part of their personalities manifest themselves after years of inhibition. Experiment also with playful face-making.

I might add that this is without a doubt one of the finest facial exercises for beauty that there is! When you break past those inhibited "ugly" emotions which you pack around behind masks, your true spirit can express itself, both through your face and especially through your eyes. Once you've gotten out your repulsions, you can go totally into your feelings of warmth, love, acceptance, softness, and radiating magnetic expansiveness.

b. Eye Warm-ups

I'd like to introduce an acupressure massage technique which is the main preventive visual exercise being done daily throughout the People's Republic of China. Twice a day in that nation, students, clerks and most factory workers pause for fifteen minutes while relaxing music is piped in, do exercises that are aimed at reducing diseases caused by tension, poor physical fitness, etc. I do not approve of having the government order everybody to do exercises, but I hope that in our freer system we can develop programs which focus on preventing diseases before they can develop, through such exercising on a regular basis. I would like to see a group of professional preventive-disease experts go to factories, offices, and schools once or twice a day and lead students and workers in particular preventive-disease

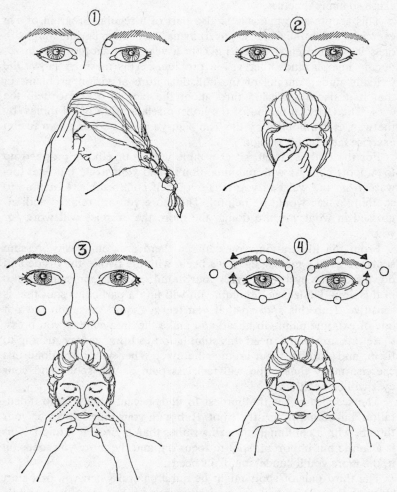

Acupressure

exercises and in meditations which would reduce the tensions that cause so many illnesses.

This acupressure massage is also part of a regular program of eye exercises which the Chinese government has been experimenting with on school children. Reports indicate a very high success rate in reducing myopia and other vision problems. This massage shows the Oriental understanding of the holistic nature of vision problems in that it deals with tension throughout the face in order to help the eyes. The Oriental notion of the holistic relationship of all things, by the way, is symbolized by the Tao sign you will be using as a fusion exercise later in this session.

For the exercise itself, sit at a table with your elbows propped up to support you. As with palming, don't bend your neck, but lean forward from the waist as you make yourself comfortable. Listening to soothing music would be helpful. The more you are relaxed and engrossed in what you are doing, the more the exercise will work for you.

From the illustration, you can see there are four basic pressure spots we will be massaging. Let's begin with the two to the inside and down from the eyebrows. With your thumbs, massage in small circles in this area. Under each thumb, you will find a particular spot that is sensitive. Rub this spot so that you feel a "sour" sensation but not one of extreme pain. Go ahead and make the area ache as you press; these pressure points need this stimulation to bring energy rushing to them, and through them around the eyes. When you have done this exercise many times, you will feel less pain on the spots, and your eyes will be healthier.

The second spot is the hardest to find, because there is no indentation, but rather a "gristly" spot. Rub with your index finger or your thumb, with a continual squeezing rather than a circular motion. This is a subtle but important spot to focus on, and the more you focus on it, the more you'll "understand" its needs.

The third pair of spots might be quite painful when you first start working there. You will use your index fingers, but place your middle fingers beside your nostrils at first, to get your index fingers the right distance from your nose. Having your thumbs support your chin is also helpful for positioning. These two spots are right beside your cheekbones and should be rubbed in circular motion with the index fingers. If you're very sore here while rubbing, it means this is a major blockage spot of energy for you, and you should promise yourself that you will give the spots regular attention until the pain lessens and moves into positive energy feelings when you rub.

The fourth massage position actually deals with six pressure spots of importance to the eyes. Put your thumbs on your temples, curl the four fingers of each hand, and rub outward across these spots with the second-joint flat area of your index and middle fingers. Do the top four spots a few times, then the bottom two, and then repeat the process a number of times.

Do remember to breathe and blink while doing these. As you experience pain in these spots your natural tendency will be to inhibit your breathing and tense against the pain. But don't do that, and you will have remarkable success with the exercise.

Once you are finished with the exercise (ten minutes or so), you will possibly experience clearer vision as you blink and look around you. This exercise is a good finishing exercise after doing exercises that work the eye muscles directly. I substitute it for part of my palming time often, because it is so important.

c. The Main Event – SEQUENTIAL VISUALIZATIONS

This "sequential" step will be helpful as you visualize. Doing visualizations regularly is important, and here is a variation in the basic visualization exercise you did earlier.

For instance, in the "tropical island" visualization, when you are watching a boat sail by, visualize a large schooner or other boat sailing past on the horizon. Allow this large boat to sail past your vision, big enough and close enough to be perfectly clear.

When it is gone, imagine another identical schooner coming by, but this one is a little farther away than the first. However, it is just as clear. Palm and breathe deeply and relax and just enjoy the sequential visualization of more and more boats going by, each one getting a little farther away from you but each one staying clear in your imagination. Stay aware of the blue of the sky and the water against the white sails of the boats. If you want, you can imagine smaller and smaller types of sailboats going by rather than having the boats get farther in the distance. Or have each boat be a different color, to add variety.

If sailboats aren't your fancy, what is? Some people imagine going for a stroll through a garden and noting a different flower or plant with each breath. Each plant that comes along should be smaller or farther away than the last, to give your imagination's eye a good

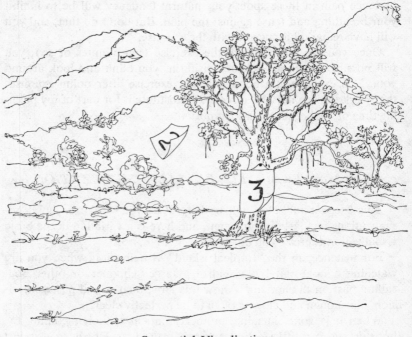

Sequential Visualization

workout. Another suggestion is different sizes, shapes, and breeds of animals. I know one person whose favorite visualization is lying at the local nude beach watching each new sunbather arrive!

A visualization which helps my eyes the most is a "number" sequential visualization. Imagine you're in a beautiful spring meadow far away from any tension or activity, sitting on a small knoll with a slight breeze blowing across the meadow. Your gaze falls on a tall tree standing in the middle of the meadow, and on the trunk of it is a pad of paper which you can see quite clearly even though it's at a distance.

On the first page of the pad is the number 1, or the letter A, whichever you prefer. Breathe and sigh gently as you look at the letter or number. Then a little breeze comes up and blows that paper away and you can see a 2 or a B on the pad, perfectly clearly. The number or letter is painted in deep black against clear white, and as the wind continues to slowly blow the pieces of paper away, the numbers or letters become smaller as they disappear, until when you get to Z or 30, the numbers are very tiny but still perfectly clear.

Adjust this visualization if you are farsighted, of course, to suit your needs. Make up anything you like!

IN BETWEEN

Since we discussed acupressure massage in this session, I'd like to include also "foot reflexology" as part of your over-all vision program. The theory of foot reflexology is that the bottoms of the feet have spots which correspond directly with parts of the body. One of these spots is for the eyes, as shown in the illustration. As with all techniques, this is not a cure-all in and of itself, regardless of what devotees may claim; but this does not discount the genuine flashes of visual clarity some people experience after a foot massage. I feel certain that foot reflexology does work to help the eyes to better health and clarity. Also, I have yet to find a person with poor vision who was not sore or tender on the visual spots of the feet. Conversely,

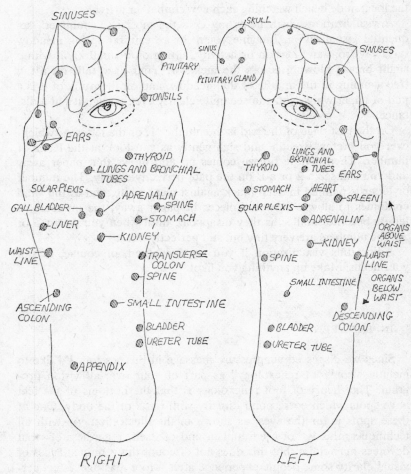

Foot Reflexology

people with good vision almost never feel any pain when this area is massaged.

You can either have someone give you a foot reflexology massage or you can work on the spots yourself. Rub firmly and deeply on the area marked on the chart for eyes, making deep circular movements while breathing into any pain you experience, and remaining aware of how this massage is affecting your vision.

I've also included on this chart the spots that are connected to other organs and parts of your body, if you want to get more fully into foot reflexology.

YOUR EYELOGUE

Write down your television-viewing habits. How often do you watch TV (hours a day on the average)? How close do you sit to the screen? Do you stare at the screen, or edge the objects being projected on the screen to keep your eyes moving? Do you watch TV with or without your glasses? Do you sit looking up at the TV from a low position, or straight-on with your chin down? Can you incorporate eye exercises into watching TV?

There is growing evidence that the radiation emitted by television, especially older color sets, is dangerous to health. Arguments range over a safe level of tolerance to this radiation, but the truth is that the radiation is there, and we are all soaking it up.

However, I assume you'll be watching your share of TV, and here are some ways to use TV for vision improvement. First of all, of course, watch as little as possible—discriminate for yourself and especially your children. Sit as far back from the set as you can, and stay at an equal height with it, as most of the radiation from TV comes from the machine at a downward angle.

As you watch the screen, edge rather than stare at the image. Keep your eyes moving; if you feel you're staring off into space when you're watching TV, turn it off and palm awhile! Palm with every commercial instead of watching the ad. Also, keep a light on in the room to offset contrast. And breathe and blink!

165

Visionetics

If your eyes are myopic, try sitting without glasses right where the image becomes blurry. Keep a chair there, and see if you can't progressively move the chair back step by step gradually. Keep track of your visual progress by how far you move your chair back as time goes by.

SESSION TWENTY

a. Whole-body Exercises

I think it only fitting to end this section of the program with a fun exercise, one which plays with the energy forces and takes you completely into the reality of your own energy field. A gentle but remarkable energy-release exercise is the "energy sweep," which can safely and easily be performed by everyone. I've seen this exercise produce dramatic flashes of clear vision, cure headaches in less than a minute, and leave virtually everyone who does it in a relaxed but energized frame of mind.

If you have been doing the hand-energizer exercise you learned in Session Eleven, you have already discovered that the hands do indeed "contain" energy. This present energy-sweep exercise takes this energy and uses it, just as palming does. As with the hand-energizer exercise, it is simple and it deals in a realm of reality which is subtle and nonconventional.

This energy sweep can be done with one, two, or three persons, with three being ideal—one receiver, two givers. The givers pass their hands over the body of the receiver, up over the spine, and then slowly over the head. Once they have moved beyond the head, they flick their wrists to shake off the excess energy picked up from the receiver's body, like so many drops of water. This might sound far-fetched, but when you've done it for perhaps four or five minutes, the receiver will tell you that something definitely did happen. The sensation feels absolutely wonderful!

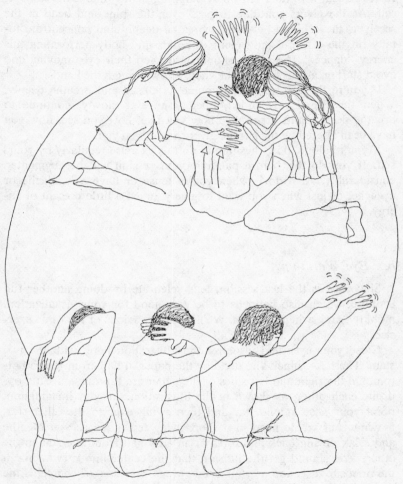

The Energy Sweep

The givers should keep their hands about an inch above the receiver's back, with their fingers overlapping slightly above the spine itself. As the givers continue to pass over the spine and head of the receiver, they should be sure to breathe deeply and concentrate totally on the graceful movement of hands and body performing this energy "dance." The givers should also keep their eyes moving and avoid staring, as this inhibits the energy flow through the hands.

If you're the receiver, keep your eyes closed and breathe deeply. When the exercise is ended, open your eyes slowly, continue to breathe deeply, and experience how you feel, how you see, how you have been altered by the gift the givers have given you.

If you're alone, don't hesitate to do this exercise regularly by yourself. If you do this before palming, your session will be augmented considerably. Also do it when you're tense or have a headache or eyeache, or just when you want to give yourself a little present of energy.

b. Eye Warm-ups

Since this is the last session, let's celebrate by doing another fun exercise, which also happens to be very good for your visualization, mobility, and swinging needs. We'll do two versions of the same exercise.

Close your eyes and visualize the illustration here, with the two stars. There is a black line dividing the paper in half from top to bottom. On the right and left sides of the paper are the stars, directly opposite each other, as shown in the illustration. In your imagination, point your nose at one star and then swing over to the other star, moving your whole head in a short-swing technique as you breathe and relax. Swing back and forth at an easy gait from one star to the other. You should get the illusion that the center line is swinging in the opposite direction as your head swings, and this, of course, is the illusion you want because it indicates you're letting go and allowing your eyes to relax.

An alternative to the "star-line-star shuttle" is the "star and moon

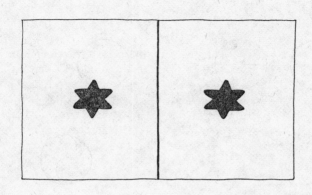

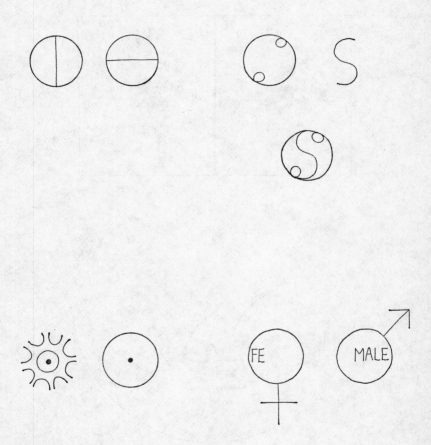

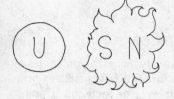

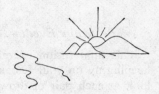

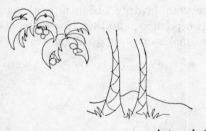

Artwork Fusion

shuttle." As in the illustration, imagine a quarter moon on its back with a star sitting in the middle. Swing your head back and forth with your eyes closed from tip to tip, and be aware that the star moves back and forth in the opposite direction. Continue shuttling for several minutes.

c. The Main Event – ARTWORK FUSION

This final fusion exercise will be relatively easy if you've been keeping up on your fusion exercises thus far. Enjoy yourself as you look at each pair of drawings, allow your eyes to focus on a point halfway in front or at a distance anywhere beyond the paper, and see what happens. In one example, the yin-yang symbol, I have also included the fused image you should get when looking at the paper in the manner you learned in the thumb fusion, in Session Fourteen.

Do remember to breathe and blink, relax, and simply allow your eyes to play with the images until they match up as a single fused picture. If this is difficult at first, don't worry, you can keep at it for as many sessions as it takes. This is such an important ability; take your time and allow your eyes to progress step by step rather than expecting them to make unrealistic leaps.

There are a number of these fusion artworks for your exercise and pleasure. Once you've done each of them several times, remember to palm and rest your eyes. Visualize your favorite fusion artwork as you palm. See if you can't see the two pictures, and then fuse them in your imagination. Also, feel free to make up your own "images" to fuse.

IN BETWEEN

You have now mastered the exercises in this vision program. If you went through the sessions quickly, you will most likely want to go back over the exercises again. If you have taken your time, and feel you have the exercises memorized and available to you without referring to the book, proceed with your own schedule. Or, if you like, take a breather for as long as you need before returning to your vision rehabilitation. We can't really force ourselves to grow faster than our natural pace, so be content with your progress and do what seems the best next step for you.

In presenting these exercises, I'm well aware that I've given you perhaps even more than you bargained for in a vision program. I hope that you've enjoyed expanding your personality and perspective while helping your eyesight. A friend of mine read this book and said somewhat jokingly, "This isn't a book about better vision, it's a book about how to attain enlightenment."

I feel that recovering clear vision is indeed attaining a very real type of enlightenment. That is why I have continued to suggest that you take your time and enjoy the path along the way. We live in the present, so we might as well enjoy the present!

I wish you a wonderful time and good success in clearing up your vision and integrating it into your personality and whole being. If we are to choose a path to greater awareness and joy, I can't think of a more direct or more enjoyable path than this one!

PART THREE

YOUR EYELOGUE

I have included in this book sample entries from the journal I kept while doing this program myself. I call the journal my "eyelogue," and I urge you to begin one now. While doing the exercises, I often found myself having sudden insights into my vision, and I began writing down my thoughts so as not to forget them. You will find that, as you spend more time thinking about and working on improving your eyesight, you will want to express your observations and reactions. I think you will find your eyelogue an invaluable learning tool in this process.

You will notice, as you read over my eyelogue, that not all my entries are positive. You, too, will have both beautiful and frustrating experiences, moments of visual clarity and emotional euphoria, and also days when you think it's all hopeless. Your eyelogue should reflect all of this. Not only will you find it a relief to be able to express your emotions and experiences, but it will be educational to turn back to early entries in the journal every so often as you progress and improve.

At certain points in the exercise program you'll find my suggestions of subjects you may want to ponder. These are effective written exercises which will help you in two ways: to reach back into your past to explore the reasons for your failing eyesight, and to reflect assertively about the environment and how it affects your eyesight as well as your over-all well-being.

For several years now, I've been teaching yoga, leading workshops for Optimal Health Associates, and in general immersing myself in the holistic health movement. I feel I've learned so much about myself and about the different paths to gaining and maintaining genuine health and mind-body integration.

However, I realize that there's a giant flaw in my life. I'm progressing as a person on many fronts as I deal with who I am and how I can realize my potential, but there's one front which I've been ignoring completely. Here I am, giving talks and leading seminars on holistic health all the time, pretending to be fairly well along the path, when all the while I'm looking out at the world through a pair of crutches.

Ugh! It's so hard to even think about me and my eyes. They are my great flaw. I know I've got to deal someday with the fact that my eyes are weak, that I'm constantly dependent on my glasses just to get around. It's frightening to think I've got to go way back and begin healing my eyes. I hate to admit, even to myself, that a part of me is so weak and messed up. But it's true. I can't deny it any longer. I want to see clearly again, without glasses!!

I don't know where to begin, but I'm sure if I keep the holistic perspective, there is hope. I guess I'll just start investigating vision retraining and follow any leads I discover.

I am armed with all the books and advice I can find on this subject. Aldous Huxley's *The Art of Seeing* is brilliant and inspiring. While I'm screwing up all my courage to come back from vision that's about 20/200 in one eye and 20/100 in the other, Huxley had the courage to start from Braille and a cane. And he made it. Not to perfect vision, as he had had a disease which permanently scarred his cornea, but to real visual independence.

Huxley's teacher was Margaret Corbett. I gather she is legendary as a vision teacher. I have several of her books, and while they don't have the literary inspiration of Huxley, they have the guidance I need now. Ah, this is one time when I wished I lived in a big city—I'd seek out a Bates teacher. As it is, I'll just have to rise to the challenge of doing it on my own.

I have a book by Bates, William Horatio Bates, who has been ostracized by the medical profession for the heretical idea that vision can be restored to its natural state. There seems no doubt that his methods do work. They apparently don't work on everybody all the time and don't restore perfect sight. It seems to depend on the individual undertaking the process. I guess that really freaks out the orthodox scientists. The human element gets them every time.

The three optometrists I've talked with all discouraged me in my quest for a path to better eyesight without glasses. They seem convinced that I can't improve my vision very much, and that it's a waste of time to do the Bates exercises. But all three of them were wearing glasses themselves, and they were really very defensive about my even wanting to get rid of my need for corrective lenses. I wonder if they've even given the Bates exercises a real try themselves? I doubt it. They make their living on the fact that people need glasses. Why would they want to come up with a way people could heal themselves and be free of glasses?

So, I'm going to start doing exercises. I've just got to jump in and start seeing what happens. Finally, I'm beginning!

Oh, hmm, ha, ha, chuckle, chuckle. Might as well laugh at myself. I've just realized I'm writing this with my glasses on. I can see perfectly well without them at close distance, and yet there they are, perched on my nose simply out of habit. Off with you!

I sit here without my glasses and look into the blur. Sigh. I don't like the way I see, not one bit. To look out into the distance is so disturbing. I get a strange sense of being off-balance, almost to the point of nausea. My chicken self wants to grab for my glasses to get rid of that blur out there.

So now I have them on. Everything's okay. But it isn't. I'm just hiding from my blur with glasses on. That blur is somehow me. Somehow, I've got to accept it, look into it, see what's there.

Now with glasses off; not trying to look into the blur, just living here in my little bubble of clarity surrounded by the blur. I have my own safe little world around me, about four feet in diameter. The rest of the world is alien, shut out by a kind of curtain. It's not so much that the rest of the world out there is fuzzy, but that there's actually a diaphanous curtain between me and reality. I'm cut off, separate.

How does that rock song go? "Break on through to the other side, break on through to the other side!"

Will I make it through the blur zone?

I've done some exercises now and they're remarkable in many ways, frustrating in others. Aha! I've caught myself with my glasses on again. God, what an insidious habit.

Howdy, blur, any word from the outside yet?

Not yet.

I palmed four times today, for about five minutes per session. It felt great to get started and accomplish a little. I'm still focused on the negative, on the fact that my mind is impatient and gets frustrated when focused on the tension I feel in my eyes. The tension did relax some, but I seem to emphasize the tension rather than the relaxation. Oh well, I'm just beginning.

On the physical level, it did feel wonderful to palm. I've been following Bates's suggestion in his book about wearing my glasses as little as possible. I went without them most of the day, and my eyes felt quite tense. When I palmed, much of that tension melted away.

I just palmed again. It gave me such a wave of relief that I almost felt like crying. I could feel the tension oozing out, somehow being absorbed by my hands. My day is made! It's a small step, my vision isn't much better. But I felt my eyes change!

I'm continuing with the Bates exercises, and also adding the yoga eye exercises I've known for years but never took seriously before. I'm amazed at how little I've thought about eyesight in the past. The more I focus on seeing, the more I realize that seeing is the most vital sense, that having it shut down and not functioning is a disaster. The body is built to work properly. What have I done to my eyes that made them go bad? That seems to be the real question.

I feel like such an uncoordinated person as I do the Bates exercises. I do my yoga postures so effortlessly, but when I go to do an eye exercise, I feel as if I don't really have any coordination in the eye muscles at all. Aha! No wonder, I've been wearing glasses for fifteen years! My eyes haven't had to do any work all that time, the glasses did the work for them, and so the eye muscles are atrophied.

More looking at myself in the mirror. I can see definitely that there is a difference between my left and my right eye. My right eye, the weakest eye, is more closed than the left eye. In fact, the whole right side of my face is stiffer than the left, having much less mobility. I even seem to talk out of the left side of my mouth.

With my eye patch on, looking around with my right eye alone is an arduous task, and the field of vision is much smaller than with the left eye.

There are esoteric schools of thought that assign the right eye with the qualities of aggressiveness, masculinity and yang, and associate the left eye with creativity, yin, feminine, intuitive qualities. If that's true, it certainly makes sense in my case.

I'm beginning to use my vision as a barometer for the rest of my feelings. If it's a bad day, I don't see well; it's that simple. What amazes me is that I never made the association before between how my eyes saw and how I felt. This seems a crucial awareness to develop and integrate.

Sometimes the exercises are a joy and fun to do. Sometimes I really get high doing them as meditations. But sometimes they're such a drag, because they make me focus on the fact that the blur is still out there. It's so hard to look right at my weakness, to accept that part of me needs help like a polio victim learning to walk.

I'm reading optometric textbooks until I'm blurry in the mind and eyes alike. I'm talking to everybody I can about vision, all aspects of it. I've learned so much; everyone has something to say about vision, except people with really bad eyesight who don't want to talk about it at all. We've got to get over this handicap barrier. People wear glasses and say they're okay, they don't want to do anything about their vision. But that's just got to be a defense against admitting they feel there's no hope for them ever improving their eyesight.

I caught myself putting on my glasses ten times today automatically, when I didn't really need them. I'd go by them, see them lying there, and put them on without thinking. But I'm learning to catch myself more and more, and I'm also learning to function without them more and more.

I used to smoke cigarettes just as I wear my glasses. Reaching for the crutch. Whew, addictions!

I'm trying to learn how to visualize a scene and it's very difficult. I mean, I can't do it, and it frustrates me. What am I doing wrong? Trying, I guess.

Took another step today, and added long swings to the palmings. I did a hundred of them, as Bates suggested, and it took only about five minutes. I felt I went through the motions correctly, but my eyes didn't seem to respond the way the book says they would. I didn't get any sense of movement, of the room swinging by in one direction as I swung in the other. What am I doing wrong?

Then, I threw the *I Ching* to get a sign from the ancients as to how this would all go. They told me:

<pre>
―――――――――   ―――――――――
―――――――――   ―――― ――――
―――――――――   ―――――――――
</pre>

BITING THROUGH changing into POSSESSION IN GREAT MEASURE

<pre>
―――― ――――   ―――――――――
―――― ――――   ―――――――――
―――――――――   ―――――――――
</pre>

I'll buy that! Especially from the Chinese. After all, China's the only country I've heard of that is instituting a nationwide preventive vision-care program. It consists of an acupressure massage done twice a day to soothing music by all students and others who do a lot of close work. They say it's working well.

I find pausing when I'm reading and looking off into the distance to be frustrating. I don't want to look up from the book, I want to stay immersed and totally shut out the outside world. I remember reading novels by the dozen back when my eyes started to go out on me. I didn't want to look up and see what was out there, I wanted to stay in my own fantasy bubble.

There was something else happening too in my reading habits. I can still feel it, that compulsion to get through the entire book, or chapter, to grasp it in its entirety before looking up. Breaking the concentration of reading seems to make me anxious, as if I'll lose it all if I don't hold on. I want time to stand still, I don't feel I can pause and go at a comfortable pace. God, I'm so compulsive, as if I'm running away from something and don't want to stop and pause and look around for fear something will be there that I don't want to see. But that's not true! I do want to see what's out there now. I want to break that bad habit and do what is good for my eyes and my psyche.

The light isn't very good tonight except directly in front of me, so when I look up the rest of the world seems encased in a furry plastic bubble. It's clear as far as my arms can reach, but then it goes blurry. Ah, but if I look at just one detail, blink and breathe, edge and breathe, there! Clearer! Wonderful!

Hey, hey! I've finally made it as a swinger! I'm starting to let the world pass me by, starting to stop hanging on to it.

I got my first sensation of movement by letting my eyes go out of focus in front of where I was looking as I swung. I knew it wasn't exactly what the books were trying to tell me, but it worked, and I most definitely got the sensation of movement. I spent about ten minutes doing that, and then let my eyes go all the way out to the right distance. The movement was not as fluid then, but it kept happening. I think it's going to keep happening more and more, too.

I imagine that the vast majority of moderate myopes could be comfortable and independent of glasses about 80 per cent of the time with just a little rethinking of what sight means and a few exercises to get the system working again. We've been given the impression that it's both a health hazard and practically a moral sin not to wear what has been "prescribed" for us. I've met countless people who were astounded to find out that there was nothing "wrong" with not wearing glasses, even though they couldn't see 20/20. They hate their glases, but have always been told they were misbehaving if they didn't wear them.

What do I think it will take to give me clear vision? Relaxed ocular muscles, relaxed ciliary muscles, coordination and agreement of eye and brain, desire to see, free flow of energy, a relaxed and accepting way of seeing what's out there, risking seeing what's out there, risking being seen by what's out there.

Total enlightenment.

Well, maybe I'll go for 20/40 instead.

I don't know if this is a good or bad step, but my frustration has won out for the time being with the purely "natural" method, and I've gone to the only optometrist I can find around here who's interested in visual training. I guess I do just still need someone to tell me what to do. What he's had to say isn't exactly thrillingly encouraging, but it's a start. At my "age" (which pretty much applies to any myope over the teen years), he doesn't think I'll be able to do much but improve one prescription level. But he's given me that level, along with bifocals so that my eyes will have to shift focus properly for close work.

I'm to wear these glasses *all the time* for the change to occur, he says. Groan. But since I'm trying it this way for a while, I'll do as I'm told. I'm also told I'll feel discomfort, and I sure as hell do. I've only had them on for an hour and I am headachy and sort of dizzy.

Is this the right way?

185

I'm getting more and more used to the glasses, but it's a mixed blessing. Wearing them so much almost did in my Bates exercising, but I believe in the exercises so much that I don't want to give them up. I think I will combine the two approaches.

The optometrist knew nothing about Bates except that in optometry textbooks he was presented as a heretical witch doctor. Next week he's going to give me some exercises to do too. If they don't incorporate anything from Bates, maybe I'll get back to adding them on my own. Finding this doctor in favor of exercises at all is a relief. I had always received one stock answer when I'd asked before: "Eye exercises won't hurt you. Eye exercises won't help you. Eye exercises will just waste your time."

I'm more used to the prescription, but not to wearing the glasses themselves. Going without just for as long as I did really made me yearn for independence from them. The eye doctor says my eyes will always need glasses since they'll never go up to 20/20. Even if they don't, every bit of time I can spend without the glasses will be a measure of independence.

I've been edging lately and having a great time at it. Just with a few days of this I can feel my eyes loosening up, and then beginning to move around with ease on their own. It's a light fluidy, free feeling. As if a great weight has been lifted (sometimes, anyway, when I'm feeling up and things are going good).

I drove Sean and a friend to the matinee yesterday, and he had to explain why I was constantly moving my head around all the time while I drove. The kid took it very matter-of-factly. Much more so than adults do. So much is frightened out of us.

Ah ha, visualization is starting to come to me. The point is not, I finally understand, to "see" an image in front of my eyes. The point is to remember and imagine in my brain. If I become really absorbed in what I am remembering I get to a point where I forget about the distinction between the darkness of my eyelids and the vividness of the memory. It's like going to a foreign film with subtitles. After a while you get so used to reading and listening that you forget they aren't speaking in English.

Hooray! It's happened. I know I'll be able to see clearly one day! I just had my first clear "flash." I palmed to a dreamy scene on a beach in Hawaii, stayed with that blissful sensation of relaxed, carefree distance vision, opened my eyes and blinked without expectation at the Snellen chart ten feet away on the wall. And, *poof,* there it was, the whole thing, crystal clear right down to the last line! A five-line jump in my visual ability. It really does work! As much as I wanted it to and hoped for it to happen, deep down I was so afraid it never would happen. But, as they say, seeing is believing!

Whew, I'm so elated. In fact, I think it was my elation that made the image blur back to "normal" after about ten seconds. I was so surprised and excited that I began to laugh and cry out, and that seemed to do it in for the time being. But I've done it once, and I'll do it again, and I'll keep doing it until it stays that way!

The first flash has been followed by two more. These times I kept on blinking and breathing and was able to hold the image for about twenty seconds. I also shut my left eye for a while to see if the right eye was doing it too, and, lo and behold, it was. From 20/200 to awfully close to 20/20!

In her book *Self-Hypnosis in Two Days,* Freda Morris grabs me with the phrase "The imagination is the prime force initiating everything we accomplish."

It's all in the way we see it inside.

There seems to be little difference, really, between the states of mind called hypnotic, meditative, alpha, and the like; from everything I've seen, they all get you to the same basic place. A place that is deeply calm, where vital energy flows, and where this energy can be allowed to heal the mind/body/soul. Getting deep inside and in tune with one's self is the key.

Let me think this all the way through: What are some of the bad things about poor vision? A bad thing about having poor vision is that it makes me dependent on artificial lenses to get by in life. Another bad thing about poor vision is that it cuts me off from other people. It also cuts me off from the reality that I could be sharing and seeing with others. It causes me physical pain and discomfort much of the time.

But I see that there's a duality to this. Let me try this one: What are some of the good things about having poor vision? A good thing about not being able to see clearly is that I don't have to take full responsibility for seeing clearly; I can be dependent on glasses. Another good thing is that I am protected against the outside world, against people and things out there that I don't want to see. Another good thing about poor vision is that it causes me pain and discomfort, and if I dwell on those I don't have to dwell on other pains and discomforts which are more far-reaching.

It's not easy to admit that I need and want many of my "problems." But it's true. Hopefully, seeing and admitting this will help me move on. Some days I am braver than others. Today I see both sides of myself.

While doing the shoulder stand and headstand I've been watching my chart and doing the yoga eye exercises. I don't feel that it's a way I'll get clear flashes, as it takes too much effort to hold the postures, but I love the rush of blood and oxygen into my eyes. Afterward they feel highly energized and ready to do more work.

It seems logically imperative that older people get upside down somehow everyday, even if it's on a slant board or just hanging over with arms and head dangling. Presbyopia seems to be simple aging, cutting down on circulation and giving in to gravity. A little reversing of gravity every day goes a long way in combating it.

Now that I'm aware of how I use my eyes during the day and what sorts of things affect the way I see, I find that certain yoga exercises really seem to give me immediate improved vision. The best seems to be the simplest, plain old stretching and yawning. The more I do these the more my eyes moisten and the tense muscles loosen up. It's always the simplest that are the best!

I also find that if I do a whole set of individual neck stretches before neck rolls that my neck is finally relaxed enough for the rolls to be really effective, and my eyes relax in complete unison with how my neck feels. I certainly do have a tense neck when I let myself get drained of energy through petty problems and overworrying about things that have to follow their own course anyway. The stiff neck goes right along with the "up tight" shoulders. I must have caught myself twenty times today holding my breath and lifting my shoulders when some little anxiety-provoking situation came up.

I don't get clear flashes from the neck and shoulder work before the exercises, but I feel that my system is much more open to letting the eyes relax. Ahhh.

I'm finding myself stuck between two "ideals" most of the time. I expect that at any moment I will become enlightened and have perfect sight thereafter. And then in other moods I sink into thinking I'll never see any more improvement. I can't imagine myself seeing any more clearly. Hello out there, middle ground, I'm lookin' for you!

I've come across a small organization called the International Myopia Prevention Association. A number of optometrists are members, but it was founded by Donald Rehm, a private citizen, who is outraged that traditional optometry is allowed to prescribe the kinds of glasses that it does for myopes. He's a firm believer in the theory that close work causes myopia and that close work done with plus lenses (the kind they give us for seeing in the distance) is what causes the further progression of the condition.

Considerable research seems to point to this being the case, though the results don't seem to be really conclusive. My O.D. agrees with this theory as well. Me, I'm in the middle. I certainly don't think that close work helps myopia, and the more you stay focused in close the harder it is going to be to come out from that. But there's so much evidence that doesn't make this *the* theory. Statistically, too many people do lots of close work without becoming myopic, to hold up the theory.

It must all boil down to *why* one wants to do close work and how much emotional stress is involved. Every theory I look at from the optometrists ignores the human, emotional factor.

My eyes are coming along faster than the eye doctor had antici-
pated (for someone my age). Hooray. I'm sure it's the addition of the
Bates work.

In fact, I feel myself really switching over to the Bates stuff again.
I hate these glasses. They have helped me make a good start, but I
can't believe that wearing glasses of any kind is going to help my eyes
much more. It's my instincts again, telling me to go natural. Back to
healing myself.

Just going to the optometrist makes me feel I'm backtracking on
my goals. Every time I go in I am overcome with anxiety. What if I
fail the test? Test? What do tests have to do with how I feel about the
way I see? Seeing as an art, as an integral part of my personality,
can't be measured on optometric instruments. The two simply contra-
dict each other. Every time I look outside myself to be told I'm okay,
I lose a big part of my okayness.

Just back from a beautiful five-day yoga retreat. Beautiful in so
many ways, yet disturbing in some others. I'd estimate that well over
half of us there wore glasses. Spiritualism is so inward, so myopic in
many ways. I'm finding that the ways I expand in yogic consciousness
do not seem to expand me within the world that I inhabit during this
lifetime. Yoga gives me great peace, but seems to compound my
aloneness and introspection. I sense other paths to the same place
opening to me somewhere. Where?

I'm giving up on my goal of 20/20 vision. It's a giving up of a part
of my ego. A neurotic, needy part. It's much more important to me to
live with myself in harmony with the way I am than to be driving for

191

an externally imposed goal. I don't give a damn about all those charts and letters. I just want to be comfortable with my sight, my vision, myself.

The goal is not to see clearly, but to relax, to let go of all the things I thought I had to see. Just to relax and see what is really there after all, which may have little to do with what I have been trying to see.

There seems to be something very important in the back of my mind, related to art and vision. I have always had certain blocks which kept me from being able to look at something, and then draw it on paper. When I'm edging, I become aware that at certain spots along a curved line I run into strange difficulties in continuing along that line—and it's the same trouble I'd have if I were trying to draw it. Something does not function. Well, I'm going to tackle this problem head-on and start drawing ten minutes a day as part of my exercises.

My trouble is that, like all myopes, I have trouble not being able to do something perfectly the first time. I'm afraid to fail, so I don't spend time working at what I can't do well. Maybe through working on my drawing patiently, without expecting myself to do anything perfectly at all, I can make progress in both my vision and my art.

Ah, I just drew one of my shoes. It doesn't look at all bad. It's not a Van Gogh, but it's a hell of a lot better than I expected it to look. I just did my edging on paper as I did it with my eyes. Is art that simple? I really want to talk about vision with some artists!

I've read that some people become farsighted, hyperopic, when they go into the Army or to college. I'd always assumed that hyperopia was something only older people got, but it seems that isn't the case. So not everybody reacts to frightening situations with myopia or astigmatism. Some people react with good old-fashioned resentment and anger, creating the symptoms that lead to hyperopia. Very interesting.

Also, I've been reading a study about policemen who become nearsighted in middle age, when they are retired to desk jobs. Do their eyes go nearsighted through strain of desk work, or are they burying anger at being tucked away at a desk job, or fear that their desk job indicates they're beyond their prime, facing old age and death?

And in my own case, becoming nearsighted as a teen-ager when I didn't want to see my environment. I wanted to be invisible, and I think I at least partially succeeded. However, the price I had to pay for invisibility was my eyesight.

I've arranged for a Bates teacher from L.A., Janet Goodrich, to come up here and give a weekend workshop. There'll be twenty of us participating. Finally, I'll get to see if I've really gotten the gist of all this right or not.

As a group, we're pretty excited about the possibilities. I hope we don't high-hope ourselves out of a good experience. After all, it's still going to be up to us, she's no magician. However, the information she sent on herself looks varied and fascinating, for sure, though. The most intriguing part is that she is a trained neo-Reichian therapist. What's that? I guess we'll find out.

The workshop with Janet was wonderful. I learned a great deal and was comforted to be reassured that I was basically right on in my directions.

The most significant thing for me was that as Janet watched me as I wore my glasses at certain times, she asked me why I did so—since I didn't really need them. Something clicked inside me. I don't need them. I guess I wanted someone I trusted to tell me so. I would like that conviction to have come first from myself, but I'll accept my need for assurance. I took them off and haven't put them back on at all except to drive. Maybe I'll never wear my glasses again.

The Bates method combined with other disciplines Janet uses is soothing, hypnotic, energizing, and completely positive. And we reacted in kind. Everyone saw better. There were some wonderful clear flashes, one particularly dramatic one complete with tears and cries of "I can see! I can see!"

I'm still not completely clear as to who Wilhelm Reich was, but I know that he was deeply involved in energy flow, life-force flow. And that he was so threatening a figure in this country that his books were burned, and he died in a federal penitentiary.

I hadn't worn my glasses for about a week and a half; just didn't have any need for them. Then I drove into town in the traffic and to a show. So, back on they went. Ugh. Everything is so artificially etched, so sharply distorted. I don't like it a bit. I can't believe that all these years we let ourselves just follow orders to "get used to the glasses" when the effect was so unnatural.

I'm finally accepting the way I see. Maybe going beyond that to loving it. I love my blur. I wonder if that is a good or a bad sign. Maybe I don't want any farther out. I'll wait and see. In the meantime I see in what I like to think of as grainy, oriental tones. Soft, flowing textures and colors. It's truly beautiful. I'd like to come up with some glasses for normal-sighted people so they could see what they are missing. There's another world beyond detail, and it's gorgeous.

Of course, reality reminds me that I'm very glad to have my artificial crutches when I need the detail.

The school system is letting me organize an adult education class in vision improvement. I'm proud of them for their pioneer spirit. It may vanish once they realize how radical the Bates method is considered by optometrists, but I'll worry about that later. Meanwhile, I can spread what I've learned, see how others respond and, no doubt, learn from those I'll be working with.

I'm in the second week of not wearing glasses at all. And I'm becoming aware of an occasional sense of strain, fatigue and frustration. I'm going to start carrying my glasses in a nice strong case so I'll be able to pop them on now and then. I think I've gone a little overboard going so cold turkey. There are times when trying to see well is too much of an added strain on top of other things going on in my life. I could get by now without my glasses if I have to—that's coming a long way from thinking I'd fall off a cliff!—but I don't think there's anything wrong with controlled use of them, as with any other drug that sometimes makes it easier to bridge the gap between me and reality.

If I wear a patch over my better eye I still have some trouble with the world swinging by completely freely. But with both eyes or the good eye alone, I am now able to let it go effortlessly. What a thrill! I not only see better afterward, but I feel so free and relaxed.

I'm through with hanging on! (Well, more and more all the time.)

I tossed a ball with Tracy for half an hour yesterday, and not only did we have a good social time, but we both had flashes of better vision, which were exciting. I continue to be surprised that doing something that's fun can help me. But it certainly makes sense that enjoyment goes hand in hand with vision improvement.

I've been thinking about "curing" my vision. Once I get my eyesight to where I like how I see (and I'm determined to do just that) will I be cured, will I just forget about my eyesight from then on out?

I don't think so, I think that me and my eyes are going to be close friends long after this team effort of vision improvement is over. What am I after anyway, in wanting to get "cured"? I'm really wanting to establish a lifelong relationship with my eyes, to become one with them in a very real sense, to stay in touch with them deeply. The last thing in the world I want is to get "cured" visually and then never do another of the vision exercises again.

I just met with my first group of eye students. It's all so exciting! I discovered that I'm not the only one with a deep conviction that the professional attitude toward vision is really lacking something. Everyone in class believes their eyes can get better. Even those who hadn't heard of Bates immediately bought tension as the cause of their problem. We shared our vision histories and found so many same or related experiences. Most of us are moderate myopes, seeing around 20/70 to 20/200. Several people have 20/20 vision but know that quality is lacking; they're a real delight to have around. Also delightful are the older people who feel strongly that the only reason they are wearing glasses is because they were always told they would have to. They have wonderful spirits. It's sure nice not to be in this alone any more.

The books by Laura Huxley and Kriyananda have me thinking about meditating on energy and energy flow. But they talk about it in general; I want to develop meditations that are specifically for the flow of energy through the eyes. Where to start? Just meditating on what I feel in my eyes for a starter. Do I feel any energy there at all, is there any pulsing flow?

Yes, but I seem mostly aware of the blockage of energy in my eyes. The tightness. So I'll meditate on the tightness, and imagine the blocks dissolving and letting the energy flow.

I've been doing the energy sweep on myself, both to help clear up my eyesight and to help clear up headaches. It does work, usually, when I concentrate and give myself to the exercise. I'm so powerful, really, why don't I just go ahead and take responsibility for that power, allow myself to heal myself? I guess I was just conditioned from birth to let the doctors take the responsibility for my health. But all they took responsibility for was my sickness, not my health. They were only interested in me when I was sick, when they could treat an illness. I want the opposite. I want to help myself, first of all, and I want to help myself stay healthy, not just help myself get well. It's such a small change in perspective, but it is really a revolution!

Today I visited the Radix Institute, which I found in the Yellow Pages under "Eye Training." It is founded and headed by a man named Charles (Chuck) Kelley, who, from what I can tell so far, believes vision problems to be purely emotional in origin. It's not just random anxiety causing random problems, but specific emotions resulting in specific manifestations. Fear, he says, is at the root of nearsightedness, and anger is at the bottom of farsightedness. He even has the personalities of myopes and hyperopes on a chart. I had to admit that I fit the myopic type perfectly.

Kelley, too, is a myope. His vision was 20/200 in one eye and 20/400 in the other. Before long that changed to 20/70. Then 20/40, where he has remained for about twenty-some years now. He was a Bates teacher and then studied and worked with Wilhelm Reich. Here's this Reich character again. Suddenly he seems to be a major figure in psychology. Why didn't I learn about him in college? I have the distinct feeling I've stumbled on something very radical.

Tomorrow I'll go back for a one-day introductory workshop and find out what this is all about.

Well, I've certainly found out what they are up to at Radix. They're even worse than the common-garden variety "touchy-feely freaks" that my father is always talking down. Not only are they touchy and feely, but they scream. The Radix people are affectionately known by their neighbors in the building as the "Screamers." I look in the Yellow Pages, and I end up affiliating myself with the Screamers! Me, who *never* screams. Never so much as raises her voice. Who visibly cringes at the sound of loud voices. . . .

Me. I screamed. And I cried. I screamed and cried in front of fifteen total strangers.

And I loved it!

I haven't felt this good, in, well . . . well, maybe I've never felt this way before. I feel so open and clear.

And my eyes. Flashes! Three perfectly clear flashes during the afternoon. But even more amazing was the clarity of the world afterward, not so much in terms of details but in terms of freshness. The world looked as if it had been freshly washed, perhaps because I feel clean and washed myself. The connection between my eyes and my emotions is completely obvious to me now. When I freed and cleansed my emotions, the same thing happened to my eyes. What an exquisite sense of freedom.

Radix. It's Greek for "root." I seem to have stumbled onto the root of the matter.

I'm tickled that this fusion work is so important because it's great fun. My first five sessions or so tired my eyes a lot and didn't seem to accomplish much in terms of my eyes responding. Then, voilà, I got the hang of it. My eyes can hold phantom images for as long as I want without any trouble. I can also move around and spread apart my targets and still keep the desired images. Gives me a great sense of strength and mobility.

The basic Bates string fusion is important because it emphasizes stretching vision, getting it out into the distances it's unused to. I have even more fun with the optometric fusion exercises, though, or at least with the versions of them I'm coming up with on my own. I love taking two halves of an image and fuse them into one. I also enjoy changing my focus at will, creating phantom images by looking in front of or behind an object or person. I can give someone a "third eye" just by focusing halfway toward the face in front of the eyes! There are even some games I learned as a kid that are great fusion exercises. The "hot dog" is the main one. You put your index fingers together at the tips, focus halfway in front of them, and there emerges this amazing little hot doglike finger with fingernails at each end. As you move your fingers apart the little one stays suspended out there in space. I like to wiggle the ends now and then. Whew, I'm really getting silly with all this!

Several people in class already have weaker prescriptions, mostly with bifocals, too. My suspicions have proved correct: They are not going through the unpleasant physical sensations I suffered, because they are already doing the relaxation exercises and relieving the strain.

One woman had a particularly bad week of being very tense without glasses. I wish she had worn them instead. It only causes guilt and strain not to wear them if it feels bad. I think this has convinced her that for her a weaker prescription would be a better first step. Also, only taking them off in easy, comfortable situations.

I've taken a closer look at my posture and have to admit that while it looks pretty good in general, it has a lot more problems than I'd thought. I've always been aware of the tension in my chest and shoulders and my tendency to stand with locked knees to hold up continually weak-feeling legs. When I study Chuck Kelley's chart on myopic traits, I have to admit that, yes, I also carry around a lot of chronic tension in my throat, jaws, scalp, and the back of my neck. I also carry my shoulders forward and my jaw rather rotated forward so that my forehead is pushed back. Optometrist Ray Gottlieb, who uses a combination of the Bates method and posture realignment, impressed this on me when he held me by the base of the skull and the jaw and lifted me into proper alignment.

Oh, triumph of triumph, I've found my anger! At least I've touched on it, admitted that I have it, and, by God, it feels tremendous. Tremendously good. Now I realize that I don't have to take out my past anger on anyone, and that I don't really have to blame anyone for anything. But it is my right to feel real, justified feelings of anger and resentment, regardless of the circumstances. When I have been violated and don't allow myself to feel the anger, I just end up burying it and turning it on myself.

I worked this through, quite literally, in a marathon fifteen-minute towel-pounding session. I let shouts and words come out at everyone and everything that had ever made me feel thwarted. During the first half of the time I was just going through the motions, but then real emotion took over. And poured out. Afterward, no headache, no guilt, just a clean free feeling . . . and . . . more of an ability to love those who mean the most to me. By not allowing myself to see my negative feelings I was squashing my positive ones as well.

My first inkling of why my right eye might be so weak came when Laura DiNuccio, a Radix teacher, made the comment that she too had such a problem and that all she really knew was that it has been speculated that the left eye is associated with feminine and creative qualities while the right eye is linked to aggressive and masculine characteristics.

Now, I read in *The Body Reveals,* a totally fascinating book by Ron Kurtz and Hector Prestera, that "sidedness" is common and significant. Not just in the eyes but in the whole body. Yes, as I examine myself more closely, it's obvious that I carry the vast majority of my tensions on my right side. All my chronic tension in my neck and back is on the right side. In my face it's much more than my eye that shows tension. The whole right side of my face is tight and frozen compared with my left side. It's so obvious once I look closely in the mirror, yet I'd just never looked closely before.

I found a table on right- and left-eye characteristics in *The Body Reveals* to peg me just as had Chuck Kelley's on myopic personality traits. The right eye manifests the ego, social relationships, distrust and paranoia, the "doing" side of one's nature and such things. Yes, I'm more of a thinker than a doer. Yes, my relationship with my father and his showing me my role in the world was impaired, since my parents were divorced when I was two. Ah, yes.

Today I feel amazed at the power of my mind/body/emotions to manipulate my view of the world to that which suited my needs. There was so much I didn't want to see. And I protected myself.

Soon after my last trip to Radix I remembered Nana. My grandmother lived with me from the time I was brought home from the hospital. I can hardly remember her at all even though I was fourteen when she died. I've realized that I can't remember her because I shut out the sight of her dying over a period of several years. She must have been a very important and positive influence in my growing up, yet I've blocked it all out because I couldn't stand to see her sitting there in the living room like a vegetable. Two strokes. My mother going to pieces under the strain. Me freezing up, withdrawing.

I got my first pair of glasses two months after her first stroke.

Now that I've discovered Radix, I've also found that other holistic approaches to emotional and physical growth can affect vision. The Radix Vision and Feeling program and a part of what goes on at the Gestalt Center in New York are the only places I know which have specific vision programs, but others report improvement as an added side effect to their work.

The Alexander method of postural restructuring appears to have helped many people, with really profound effects if the students are young enough. Other straight body-work methods like Rolfing and Postural Integration report some success too. Posture obviously has a lot to do with it, especially for us myopes. I even see better after going to the chiropractor.

I feel that the best methods are those that integrate emotional and feeling growth with body work, programs such as Radix and bioenergetics. But, obviously, anything which deeply affects and changes an individual toward being more open and self-secure can change vision as well.

I've discovered something strikingly similar in many of the people in class with astigmatism and fusion as their main problems. Almost without fail those who experience visual discomfort rather than blurred vision carry their heads, and often their whole bodies, way off to one side. The brain, then, is just having to strain so much to put together the imbalanced picture that it's getting.

When I work with these people on aligning their spines, they experience even more of a sense of exhilaration, relief, and relaxation than the rest of us, or so it seems. It will take a lot more time watching people and working with them to see if this is a really valid point, but it feels very right.

I'm finding the process of learning the art of seeing to be very much like learning music. My first attempts at both arts were so clumsy and painful, I didn't know if I would ever get the hang of it. My fingers wouldn't respond to the guitar fretboard, and similarly, my eye muscles just sat there frozen. Ease and spontaneity seemed so far off. And now, now I can change chords in music effortlessly and do the same with my eyes from near to far. What ease, what spontaneity! Whoopee!

This pause to reflect has been invaluable. I didn't even realize how far I had come until I reread my journal for the first time. Baby, you have come a long way and it feels great.

I've received a packet of books, pamphlets, and tapes from the Cancer Counseling and Research Center in Fort Worth, Texas. Now here are doctors up to some amazing stuff! Dr. Carl Simonton and his wife, Stephanie, have begun a program of counseling and meditation for cancer patients who have reached the stage where all hope of a medical cure or arrestment has been given up. And lo and behold, with a program of visual meditation many of these terminal patients are living far, far beyond their forecast times, and some have had tumors completely disappear. What a relief to see that the medical community is leaning toward seeing the mind and body as one. Think what they'll do to cancer when they start using this program before the patients are deemed terminal!

Just as Kelley and others are finding personality types that lend themselves to certain vision problems, the Simontons and others are finding the same thing with cancer. It seems that certain personalities get certain cancers and all of them tend to share the common problems of inhibited life-styles, being unable to grieve fully over the loss of loved ones, depression, and a general lack of ability to express emotions. Sounds like most of us. No wonder it gets one out of four. And heart disease gets one out of three. And vision problems get one out of two.

❧

The retina of the eye is so amazingly complex. Scientists can't imagine ever really understanding it. It's also so beautiful in photographs. Gorgeous shades of orange and yellow. The macula, where the clear vision happens, is a brilliant yellow sun surrounded by the orange of the rest of the retina.

I've seen pictures, too, of retinas in very bad shape. High myopes have them all stretched out of proportion, the coloration is often different. I can see why the scientists can look at them and say how in the world could they ever get back into proper shape. Stretch marks after childbirth are nothing in comparison. And yet it happens, I know it does. I've been there when high myopes have experienced medically unaccountable clear flashes.

As I palmed today I tried to envision the retina of my eyes. To relate to the very literal part of my brain that lives right there. All those intricate layers. It's an odd one to dwell on. I don't have any feeling of sensation or emotions attached to it.

❧

I think I've found perhaps my most powerful healing, palming meditation. I combined the visualization techniques used by a team of doctors in Texas to treat cancer with the idea of healing my eyes. I visualized my eyes in almost a cartoonlike state, surrounded by bands of muscles. I could see how much more tightly bound down the right one was.

Three phases of the meditation. One is breathing energy in and out. I can visualize it as a solid warm flowing force, of silver now, seeping into the eyes and their muscles as I inhale. The energy stretches and enlarges the eyes, relaxing the muscles at the same time.

Then as I exhale, the muscles stay in their relaxed stretch and vibrate in warmth as the energy flows freely out the eyes.

I also use a mantra: "Soft eyes." Repeating it gently over and over again to myself as I palm and visualize the tight eyes and muscles becoming softened and relaxed from their desire to be vulnerable. Sometimes this visualization makes me cry gently. It always makes me feel good afterward.

The other variation I do is seeing the muscles around the eyes in technicolor and scope, big, hard, and tensely throbbing. Then I see my own hands come in and begin gently massaging. The massage goes as deep as I'm ready for at the time. A few times I have allowed it to go very deep, and I swear I could feel the muscles really relaxing. I felt the love I was able to give through my imaginary hands to the muscles.

APPENDIXES

THE SEVEN BASIC EXERCISE GROUPS

WHOLE-BODY EXERCISES

PALMING AND VISUALIZATION

REVISIONING AT A GLANCE:

A Program Guide

Each session contains the following sections:

  a. Whole-body Exercises
  b. Eye Warm-ups
  c. The Main Event

SESSION ONE

  a. Yawning, whole-body stretching
  b. Exploring your blur zone
  c. Palming

SESSION TWO

  a. Stretching and reverse-gravity hanging
  b. Tapping; butterfly winks; accepting your blur
  c. Edging; palming

SESSION THREE

  a. Aerobic conditioning; running in place
  b. "Seeing one thing best"; thumbnail edging
  c. Fusion, "looking through the gate"; palming

SESSION FOUR

    a. Yogic chest expander
    b. Lazy-eight, open-eye shifting exercise
    c. Short swings—"painting" swings

SESSION FIVE

    a. Progressive relaxation—the "sponge"
    b. Accommodation—"whipping"
    c. Finger-shift fusion

SESSION SIX

    a. Wake-up facial massage
    b. Talking to your blur; palming
    c. Accommodation—near-far chart; palming

SESSION SEVEN

    a. Energy release—upper-body hip rotations
    b. Picket short swings; palming
    c. Long swings; palming

SESSION EIGHT

    a. Mirror eye contact
    b. Sunning visualization
    c. Sunning—short swings

SESSION NINE

    a. Neck relaxation exercises
    b. Short swings
    c. String fusion

SESSION TEN

    a. Neck and shoulder self-massage
    b. Yoga eye exercises
    c. Scene visualization

SESSION ELEVEN

    a. Reichian breathing
    b. Eye contact after breathing
    c. Hand energizer and palming

SESSION TWELVE

    a. Sun salutation (twelve-position yoga exercise)
    b. Visualization of salutation postures
    c. Long swings; flashing; sunning; palming

SESSION THIRTEEN

    a. Grounding exercise
    b. "One thing best" counting exercise
    c. Visualization and memorization

SESSION FOURTEEN

    a. The Lowen bow
    b. Sun Sandwich
    c. Thumb fusion

SESSION FIFTEEN

    a. Woodchopper energizing exercise
    b. Dice tossing for vision improvement
    c. Juggling; frisbee

SESSION SIXTEEN

a. Yoga shoulder-stand posture
b. Solitaire for better vision
c. Healing visualization

SESSION SEVENTEEN

a. Emotional release, "towel and racket pounding"
b. Eye contact and mirror reflection
c. Patching for monoscopic vision exercise

SESSION EIGHTEEN

a. Reichian breathing, "running away" exercise
b. Pelvic rock relaxation
c. Ruler and yardstick fusion; nose writing

SESSION NINETEEN

a. Freeing the "facial mask"
b. Acupressure massage for the eyes
c. Sequential visualizations

SESSION TWENTY

a. Energy sweep exercise
b. "Star-line-star" and "star and moon" shuttles
c. Artwork fusion

SAMPLE SCHEDULES

Here are some ideas as to how you might schedule exercises into your usual life-style. The time you spend with each exercise is flexible, as you'll learn which kinds of exercises you need the most, and will want to concentrate extra time on those. The important thing to remember when designing an exercise schedule for yourself is to include an exercise from each of the seven groups. This is easy to arrange if you can break your schedule up into two or more periods. Just be sure to allow yourself an hour a day for work on your vision.

The one area of exercises not included in each schedule here is sunning, as the time you have available for exercise may not always be when and where the sun is. If you can get out into the sun for these times, so much the better. The schedules also do not include reminders to blink, breathe, and to keep your eyes moving rather than staring. These habits are so vital that you should try to do them all during the day, in addition to the fixed exercise periods.

Fit as much vision work into your days as possible. Remember, this is something you are doing because it feels good; allow yourself lots of time and good feelings.

A. *THE EIGHT-MINUTE VISION-HEALTH PLAN*

1. 2 min.: Swings
The most crucial are short swings, all variations. If possible, do them in the sun.

2. 2 min.: Centralization and Mobility
Long swings are the most important, vary occasionally.
3. 1 min.: Fusion
Any kind. Thumb fusion is the easiest and quickest here.
4. 1 min.: Accommodation
Any kind. Whipping and finger shift are quickest here.
5. 2 min.: Palming
Palm longer if possible.
Palm either to blackness or with a visualization.

B. *THE FIFTEEN-MINUTE VISION IMPROVEMENT PLAN*

1. 2 min.: Whole-body Exercise
Preferably a gentle warm-up, such as stretching and hanging.
2. 2 min.: Swings
Any variation. In sun if possible.
3. 2 min.: Fusion
Any variation.
4. 2 min.: Palming
With or without visualization.
5. 2 min.: Accommodation
Any variation.
6. 3 min.: Palming and Visualization
Any variation.
7. 2 min.: Whole Body
Something gentle but stimulating, such as the acupressure massage, foot reflexology, or neck and shoulder massage.

C. *THE THIRTY-FIVE MINUTE PLAN*

1. 5 min.: Whole Body
A good warm-up, say, stretches followed by the sun salutation.
2. 5 min.: Swings
Short swing variations, preferably in the sun.

3. 5 min.: Fusion
Any variation.
4. 5 min.: Palming and Visualization
Any variation, longer if the eyes still feel strained.
5. 5 min.: Centralization and Mobility
Long swings more often than not. Do them sometimes with one eye and then the other patched.
6. 5 min.: Accommodation
Any variation.
7. 5 min.: Palming and Visualization
Any variation.

D. *THE ONE-HOUR INTENSIVE PLAN*

1. 5 min.: Whole Body
Any variations which begin gently and then invigorating, such as stretching, followed by sun salutation or woodchopper.
2. 10 min.: Swings
Some in sun if possible, go through as many short-swing and shuttle variations as leisurely as you can.
3. 5 min.: Centralization and Mobility
Long swings are most important. I would recommend four minutes of them followed by any other variation.
4. 10 min.: Fusion
One or more variations. Stop before the time is up if your eyes get too tired.
5. 5 min.: Palming and Visualization
Any variation. Longer if necessary.
6. 5 min.: Whole Body
Preferably something energizing such as the chest expansion, pelvic rock, Reichian breathing and running.
7. 5 min.: Whole Body
Something to relax from the more energizing one, such as the sponge, wake-up massage, or neck relaxer.

8. 10 min.: Accommodation
Any variation, though the near-far chart is most recommended.
9. 5 min.: Palming and Visualization
Any variation. Take as much time as you can.

E. *THE TWO-HOUR EXTENDED PLAN*

This is similar to the one-hour plan, except you would take more time for each exercise. This would be especially helpful and important in the relaxation exercises, the whole body energizers, and with palming and visualization.

SUGGESTED READING

This listing of books is meant to help you further explore avenues that will aid you in improving your sight. Those books which do not relate directly to vision per se are mentioned so you may discover more about the "holistic" approach to health.

Achterberg, Simonton and Matthews-Simonton (editors). *Stress, Psychological Factors and Cancer*. Fort Worth, TX: New Medicine Press, 1976.

Bates, William H. *Better Eyesight Without Glasses*. New York: Holt, Rinehart and Winston, 1940.

Bean, Orson. *Me and the Orgone*. New York: St. Martins Press, 1971.

Cooper, Kenneth. *The New Aerobics*. New York: M. Evans, 1970.

Corbett, Margaret Darst. *Help Yourself to Better Sight*. New Jersey: Prentice-Hall, 1949.

Franck, Frederick. *The Zen of Seeing*. New York: Random House, 1973.

Gregory, R. L. *Eye and Brain*. New York: McGraw-Hill, 1966.

Hackett, Clara A. *Relax and See*. New York: Harper and Brothers, 1955.

Hutschnecker, Arnold A. *The Will to Live*. New York: Cornerstone Library, 1977.

Huxley, Aldous L. *The Art of Seeing*. Seattle, WA: Montana Books, 1975 (reissue of original 1942 version).

Jackson, Jim. *Seeing Yourself See*. New York: E. P. Dutton, 1975.

Kelley, Charles R. *New Techniques of Vision Improvement*. Santa Monica, CA: The Radix Institute, 1971.

—— *Psychological Factors in Myopia*. Santa Monica, CA: The Radix Institute (P.O. Box 3218).

Kraskin, Robert A. *How to Improve Your Vision*. L.A., CA: Wilshire Book Co., 1973.

Kurtz, Ron and Prestera, Hector. *The Body Reveals*. New York: Harper and Row, 1967.

Leonard, George. *The Ultimate Athlete*. New York: Viking Press, 1975.

Lowen, Alexander. *Bioenergetics*. New York: Penguin Books, 1976.

—— *The Way to Vibrant Health*. New York: Harper and Brothers, 1977.

McCamy, John and Presley, James. *Human Life Styling*. New York: Harper Colophon, 1975.

Morris, Freda. *Self-Hypnosis in Two Days*. New York: E. P. Dutton, 1975.

Ott, John. *Health and Light*. New York: Pocket Books, 1976.

Peppard, Harold M. *Sight Without Glasses*. New York: Doubleday & Co., 1940.

Reich, Wilhelm. *Character Analysis*. New York: Farrar, Straus & Giroux, 1949.

Rodale, J. I. *The Natural Way to Better Eyesight*. New York: Pyramid Books, 1968.

Rosanes-Berrett, Marilyn. *Do You Really Need Eyeglasses?* New York: Hart, 1974.

Spino, Michael. *Running Home*. Millbrae, CA: Celestial Arts, 1977.

Vishnudevananda, Swami. *The Complete Illustrated Book of Yoga*. New York: Bell, 1960.